BOVRIL, WHISKY AND GRAVEDIGGERS

THE SPANISH FLU PANDEMIC COMES TO THE WEST MIDLANDS (1918-1920)

MAGGIE ANDREWS WITH EMMA EDWARDS

Published by West Midlands History Limited
Minerva Mill Innovation Centre, Alcester, Warwickshire, UK.
© 2019 West Midlands History Limited.
© All images are copyright as credited.

The rights of Maggie Andrews and Emma Edwards to be identified as authors of this work have been asserted by them in accordance with the Copyright, Designs and Patents Act 1988.

All rights reserved. No part of this publication may be reproduced, stored in a retrieval system, or transmitted, in any form or by any means, electronic, mechanical, photocopying, recording, or otherwise, without the prior permission of West Midlands History Limited. This book is sold subject to the condition that it shall not, by way of trade or otherwise, be lent, re-sold, hired or otherwise circulated without the publisher's prior consent in any form of binding or cover other than that in which it is published and without a similar condition including this condition being imposed on the subsequent purchaser.

ISBN: 978-1-905036-64-6

Gravestone cover image: istockphoto
Caric Press Limited, Merthyr Tydfil, Wales.

Contents

Acknowledgements	4
CHAPTER ONE Introduction	5
CHAPTER TWO 'The Spanish Lady' comes to the Midlands	13
CHAPTER THREE The enemy on the home front	26
CHAPTER FOUR Bovril and whisky: everyday life during the influenza pandemic	42
CHAPTER FIVE Doctors, nurses and the challenges of providing medical care	57
CHAPTER SIX Considerable inconvenience and the business of dying	73
CHAPTER SEVEN Schools and the young	86
CHAPTER EIGHT Afterword: loss, legacies and futures	99
Sources	107
Further reading	108
Index	109

Acknowledgements

Local history projects, such as this, require the knowledge, know-how, skills, resources and time of a multitude of people and my very sincere thanks go to them all. Firstly, Mike Gibbs whose enthusiasm and financial support through History West Midlands was invaluable in facilitating a research project into this fascinating area of social history. Louise Price, curator of the George Marshall Medical Museum, successfully applied for financial support from the British Society for the History of Science for a postgraduate student, Laura Mainwaring, to work on the history of the Spanish Flu in Worcestershire. Mike Wheeler introduced Emma Edwards into the project, and she was able to provide invaluable scientific expertise. Worcestershire, Staffordshire, Herefordshire, Warwickshire, Birmingham and Dudley archives have given important help. The knowledge and skills of all who work in these archives are an invaluable resource for those studying the history of the West Midlands.

Importantly, a number of University of Worcester history students burrowed around in these archives and pored over microfiche records and computer databases to uncover many of the stories of how this pandemic shaped the lives of the ordinary people in the region; thank you Jack Edwards, Jade Gilks, Niall Herbert and Elspeth King. Thanks also go to Emmylou Field and Fintan McBride of Hanley Castle High School who undertook research for this book as part for their work experience in 2018. I hope that the skills that you have demonstrated on this project are utilised in your future careers. This book is dedicated to Worcester history students - past, present and future.

CHAPTER ONE

INTRODUCTION

'Spanish Flu' killed between 50 and 100 million people across the globe during 1918 and 1919 - more than ten times as many as were killed in the First World War. Its impact differed across the world; in Western Samoa 22% of the population died as a result of the pandemic. In Britain the death toll was regionally varied: 0.49% overall but 0.51% in the Midlands and 0.53% in the North of England. The pandemic came in three waves. The first arrived in spring 1918 and was on the wane by the middle of July: it often involved familiar symptoms, headaches, sore throat, weakness and fever with the vast majority of people recovering after a few days. However, by early autumn a new more lethal strain of the flu had been clearly identified: this lasted until the end of December, and had far more severe symptoms. Spring 1919 saw a third wave of flu, intermediate in its severity between the previous two waves. In most areas of Europe the pandemic was over by May 1919. However, there were reports of flu in Peru in 1920 and the Medical Officer of Health in Birmingham also considered that flu had returned to the city that same year.

According to the Registrar-General data in 1920, Regional Mortality Rates for influenza were as follows:

Influenza death rate each year per 1,000 of the population

	Pandemic	First wave	Second Wave	Third Wave
London	4.9	1.1	8.8	3.3
North	5.3	2.0	7.8	5.0
Midlands	5.1	1.1	8.6	3.3
South	4.3	0.8	7.6	3.1
Wales	4.3	1.5	6.6	3.5
England and Wales (all)	4.9	1.4	7.9	3.8

CHAPTER ONE

Influenza pandemics had occurred before, and indeed have happened since, but no other pandemic has had such a significant impact. During the previous pandemic, so called 'Russian' or 'Asiatic' flu of 1889-90, the chances of surviving the infection were very good. Only about 0.15% of those infected would die. The Spanish flu was a much more virulent foe, with a death rate over ten times higher, and a much higher infection rate. The Centers for Disease Control in Atlanta estimated that one in three of the global population became infected - this equates to 500 million people. The flu's impact was felt most acutely in individual families and local communities. Its influence could be seen across the West Midlands in the long queues outside doctors' surgeries and pharmacies; it was experienced in the factories that lost production, the schools and cinemas that were closed. The pandemic led to an unprecedented and unmanageable demand for undertakers' services.

The Spanish flu is now understood to have originated in Kansas in the USA, brought to Europe by soldiers sailing across the Atlantic to fight on the Western Front. It was named the Spanish Flu because the press in Spain were the first to discuss the virus. As a neutral country, Spain was not subject to the censorship that other countries experienced, and therefore reported on the progress of the illness in the country, particularly when King Alfonso XIII became unwell, quickly followed by other members of his government, including the Finance Minister and the Prime Minister. When the first cases of flu occurred in Britain, they hit a country that was war-weary after nearly four years of conflict, with little hope of an end in sight.

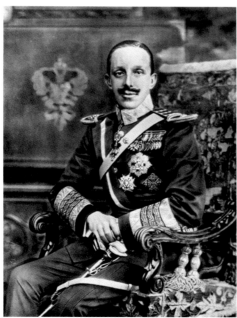

Portrait of King Alfonso XIII of Spain (1886 – 1941), original in the Museu Nacional d'Art de Catalunya

CHAPTER ONE

The Allies were having little success in their endeavours to break the stalemate on the Western Front and on 11 April 1918 the Germans were poised to re-take Passchendaele. Those on the home front were struggling to cope with the death and disruption caused by men fighting in foreign fields and zeppelin raids in Britain. Housewives battled to feed their families as a food crisis led to shortages, price rises, lengthy queues and finally the introduction of rationing in 1918. Throughout the conflict the government had increasingly interfered in the lives of ordinary citizens, introducing both conscription and progressively draconian amendments to the Defence of the Realm Acts that covered everyday activities such as pub opening hours, the strength of beer, the sale of cakes and bread and the operation of the blackout.

The West Midlands region was at the heart of the industrial production needed for the technological warfare that made the First World War so deadly. Its mines in Staffordshire and the Black Country produced coal; these areas also produced iron ore to make weapons. Factories across the region turned out

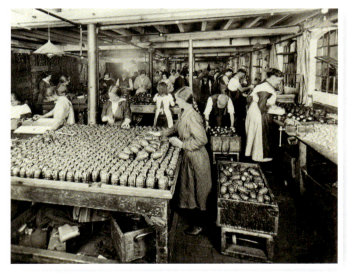

Women workers at Mills Munitions, Birmingham.

munitions: for example, at Washwood Heath in Birmingham, Rotherwas in Hereford, Blackpole in Worcester, at the Siemens engineering works in Stafford and the White or Poppe's Fuse Factory in Coventry. Likewise TNT was manufactured by Albright & Wilson at Oldbury in the Black Country and a

CHAPTER ONE

machine-gun repair factory operated at Burton-on-Trent. War production was not just about munitions, but anything and everything needed to enable the army to conduct industrial warfare: tin helmets made by Sankey's at Bilston, whistles produced in Birmingham's Jewellery Quarter and army blankets woven by the carpet makers of Kidderminster. Farms, market gardens and smallholdings grew the food needed to feed both civilians and armies; in the Evesham Vale fruit was grown to provide the ingredients needed to make the infamous plum and apple jam consumed by soldiers at the front. This wartime production had to carry on despite thousands of the region's men being absent fighting with the armed forces, some never to return. To the death toll from the battlefronts, in a little over a year, the flu virus added further deaths on the British home front, and like the war, the flu pandemic led to fatalities amongst those in their twenties and thirties. Florence, the youngest daughter of Mrs Bertha Cowley of Fladbury in Worcestershire, was a victim of influenza as the conflict reached its conclusion in November 1918. The previous year Florence's twin brother Arthur had died on active service in France. According to the local newspaper at Florence's funeral 'the grave was completely hidden from view by flowers'.

Little wonder then that in European history and memory, the devastating consequences of the influenza pandemic have often been either eclipsed by or entwined with the death and injury caused by the First World War. There were six times as many fatalities from conflict in Germany than from flu, four times as many in France and three times as many in England and Wales. In all other continents the flu was responsible for many more deaths than war and it was particularly devastating in India. In Europe, however, for many at the time, like Mr and Mrs Slade Nash of Martley, Worcestershire, influenza was yet another element of the misery and sorrow that warfare inflicted upon their lives. They had already lost two sons in the war when their daughter Margaret died from the flu in October 1918.

Whilst the First World War did not cause the pandemic, the mobility of people in wartime, shifting between countries or regions, helped spread the influenza. *The Times* noted on 18 December 1918 that once the disease reached London it radiated out through Birmingham, Nottingham and other major centres via the rail networks. All manner of public places where people gathered together in wartime: schools, factories, churches, cinemas, theatres and public transport helped to spread the virus. Influenza moved quickly between those in

CHAPTER ONE

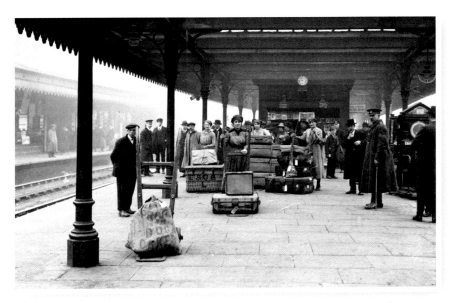

Porters awaiting trains while the passengers were inadvertently spreading flu.

close proximity to one another in the armed forces on the battlefronts, on leave, in training or POW camps or hospitals. And when men were demobilised and repatriated they became efficient carriers of the virus, the spread of which was assisted by others who were equally mobile: refugees, migrant labourers and children. Perhaps just as importantly the cultural climate of the First World War and the political priorities of the conflict shaped the attitudes and approaches to the flu and the anxieties flu evoked. It was wartime that was responsible for the lack of people with the appropriate skills to care for the victims of the influenza pandemic on the home front in the West Midlands.

Seasonal flu was a familiar phenomenon in the early twentieth century as it is now; it affected 10% of the population in the winter months and led to the death of approximately 12,000 people annually. These were usually the old or the very young for whom influenza could be a precursor to more serious illnesses, pneumonia or bronchitis, which were dangerous in an era before the use of antibiotics like penicillin. However, a unique feature of this pandemic, estimated to have infected up to a third of the British population in 1918 and 1919, was the age distribution of the deaths from Spanish flu. Many of the fatalities such as Florence Cowley were young, and they, like those who died in the conflict, were a lost generation.

CHAPTER ONE

INFLUENZA TOLL.

Birmingham Death-roll of 1,223.

LAST WEEK THE WORST.

Up to date the prevailing influenza epidemic has produced a death roll for Birmingham of 1,223. Yesterday's health returns for the city showed that the number of deaths during the past week was larger than the total of the six weeks epidemic which visited the city last summer. Whereas the latter claimed 312 victims, 381 deaths from influenza were recorded last week.

That total is almost as large as the aggregate death roll during what is known as the Russian influenza epidemic in the early nineties, when the number of victims reached 425.

The general death rate for the city last week of 43 per thousand is believed to be a record one, for something like half a century.

A Comparison.

An indication of what this means is obtained by comparing that rate with the figures for the corresponding week last year, when under normal conditions the percentage was as low as 8.2 per 1,000.

Directly and indirectly it is estimated that the prevailing epidemic was last week responsible for 500 deaths, but the actual figures for the past three weeks are as follow:—

	30 Nov.	23 Nov.	16 Nov.
Death rate per 1,000	43.0	35.6	28.5
Total deaths	717	594	475
From influenza	381	278	235
From respiratory diseases	123	130	85

The Black Week.

Yesterday Dr. Robertson, Medical Officer of Health, expressed the opinion that last week would prove the Black Week of the epidemic, but admitted that it was impossible to say definitely, as the department had no notification of the number of cases.

An inquiry at the Education Department shows an improvement, for only about 30 schools are closed, as compared with 45 a week ago.

In response to an appeal by the Lord Mayor, a conference of local medical men will be held at the Council House to-day to discuss the possibility of adopting additional measures, either to reduce the number of new cases or of dealing more effectively with patients.

Press reports told of rising death tolls, including this one in the Birmingham Gazette, *Tuesday 3 December 1918.*

Courtesy of the Library of Birmingham

Previous and more recent flu pandemics have seen the highest fatality rates among the very young, due to immature functioning of the immune system, and among the elderly, due to an age-related loss of ability to fight new strains of the virus. This pattern is a characteristic of flu, both pandemic and seasonal, and explains the vaccination policies of many countries, which prioritise the young and the old. Spanish flu was different in that it disproportionately affected younger adults, the peak age of death was 28. For example, between 1914 and 1917, on average 118 people per year between the ages of 20 and 45 died from influenza in London. In 1918 that figure rose to 5890, giving a fifty-fold increase in the death rate. These were supposedly the strongest, fittest people, with mature, but not elderly immune systems. They should have been the best equipped to fight off the infection but they were not. Amongst other age groups there was a fourteen-fold increase in deaths in 1918 compared to the three previous years. The reasons for these phenomena are still

CHAPTER ONE

being explored, but there are some interesting theories, backed up by meticulous laboratory research.

The first is that it was the strength of the immune response itself that proved fatal. The powerful immune responses of young adults, instead of just killing the virus or virus-infected cells, damaged healthy tissues. This made the patients more susceptible to secondary, bacterial infections, which could prove fatal. This over-reaction by the immune system is known as a 'cytokine storm', cytokines being chemical messengers that cells of the immune system use to communicate with one another. An immune cell, on recognising a threat, produces cytokines, which tell other immune cells to respond to the threat. Research has shown that the 1918 virus was capable of stimulating this phenomenon in people. The virus was also capable of replicating not just in the airways like normal flu, but in other parts of the body. This meant that the over-reaction of the immune system could be experienced throughout the body.

There is also a hypothesis that younger adults were far more geographically mobile and therefore more likely to be exposed to bacterial strains that they had no prior immunity to. This phenomenon is still seen every September when thousands of young adults move to new towns for university and are likely to come down with what has been nicknamed 'freshers' flu'. These bacteria may have acted as a secondary infection that ultimately proved fatal for the young people who caught influenza. There is some evidence that recent arrivals in army barracks were more likely to die than troops who had been stationed there for some time. However, this hypothesis is almost impossible to test, and it may never be known what contribution the mobility of populations or secondary infections played in the final death toll.

Another novel feature of the Spanish flu was its symptoms. Typically, at the time, flu was seen as a 'three-day fever' with the patient improving after it had run its course. Lethargy, aches and pains, the headache that worsens when you move your head, are features most of us are familiar with. The 1918 flu was much more severe, with the most severe symptom, which doctors at the time recognised as an indication the patient was in grave danger, being heliotrope cyanosis. This involved patients' skin and lips becoming a purplish blue colour. A doctor by the name of Hubert French, in a report for the Ministry of Health in 1920, estimated that 95% of patients with this sign died. It is now thought to have been caused by a lack of oxygen. Damage caused by the virus, or

CHAPTER ONE

secondary infections, resulted in the tissues of the lungs leaking fluid into the small air sacs of the lungs, meaning the patients struggled to absorb sufficient oxygen when breathing.

During the early twentieth century, doctors still had very few clues about what was causing which disease. Nowadays when patients attend a GP surgery, they are frequently told that 'it's just a virus': the symptoms are so similar, and the disease course mild, there is not really a lot of point determining the exact cause. However, when it is clinically useful, modern medicine can often identify the exact virus or bacteria responsible. This was not an option during the Spanish flu, so it was almost impossible to determine exactly which pathogen was responsible. This led to difficulties in determining exactly what the patients had died of, and consequently in determining exact figures for the number of deaths due to influenza.

For a period of a little over a year the population of the West Midlands lived with this uncertainty, coupled with anxiety, panic, rumour, the fear of death, sorrow and grief caused by influenza. Some experienced psychosis, miscarriage and other longer-term consequences of perhaps the worst pandemic the world has ever seen. Birmingham was one of the first cities to be associated with Spanish flu. On 22 June 1918 *The Times* noted: 'Birmingham was the first provincial city to experience a sudden and sustained rise in influenza mortality with deaths also occurring in neighbouring Wolverhampton and Coventry at the same time.' Only a few days later, Colin Priestman's mother in Birmingham received a letter from her son, who was working with an army convey in France informing her: 'We are going through an epidemic of influenza on the convey. At the moment there are seven of us in bed with it, and amongst them myself. One case was quite recovered, but this afternoon another quickly succumbed to the "grippe" and has taken the vacant bed.' For many people, news that those in the armed forces were also in danger added to a growing awareness of the spread of influenza on home front. The chapters that follow draw upon a serendipitous array of sources, letters and newspapers, diaries, Medical Officer of Health Reports, oral histories and adverts to explore experiences and stories of ordinary people during the Spanish flu pandemic in the West Midlands. These stories, particularly in the first chapters, are intermingled with contemporary scientific understandings of influenza which often illuminate how difficult it was to control the pandemic 100 years ago.

CHAPTER TWO

'THE SPANISH LADY' COMES TO THE MIDLANDS

Many of those who encountered the pandemic of 1918 had memories or had heard family stories of the Russian Flu of 1889 – 1894. The prior pandemic had claimed approximately 1 million lives in its three waves, the second of which was the most severe. Reports from the *Worcester News* on 11 January 1890 explained that:

> The malady, which is now known as the Russian Influenza has at length gained a footing in Worcester. The influenza first made its appearance several days ago, when a gentleman at one of the banks in the city became ill and in the course of time developed undoubted symptoms of influenza. Since then the outbreak has rapidly spread, and there are nearly two hundred cases in the city and suburbs.

The report continued to explain that rich and poor alike were falling victim to influenza and that although no one had yet died there were cases in Kidderminster, Stourport, Pershore, Bromsgrove and Evesham. It took a long time for people to realise how much more virulent and dangerous the Spanish flu was; indeed initially in 1918 the seriousness of influenza was often underestimated.

An awareness that the region was in the grip of a pandemic came slowly to the West Midlands. During the late spring and early summer months, the managers of munitions and iron works, mines and transport operators began to observe significant levels of absenteeism and even people collapsing at work with influenza. The *Birmingham Daily Mail* gave an account on 28 June 1928 that: 'Work people in many factories have been stricken with the complaint, and at one large works alone several hundreds of people are absent.' In an era where there was no sick-pay, no worker stayed away from work lightly. Such a decision carried financial hardship and threatened their often precarious family finances, sometimes irreparably. Nevertheless the following day it is clear influenza was threatening war production, and the newspaper related how:

CHAPTER TWO

At one large works in Hales Owen district, where 5,000 hands are engaged, between 700 and 800 are away; while at some of the smaller works so many of the employees are affected that it has been found necessary to close down certain departments for a week. Hundreds of operatives have collapsed and been removed to their homes in motor ambulances and other vehicles.

Dr Robertson, the Medical Officer of Health in Birmingham in writing his report at the end of the 1918, was quite clear that in this wave of influenza 'the onset was usually sudden and alarming - the prostration severe. In four or five days most of the patients were at work or school again.' However, at the start of the pandemic, there was a degree of uncertainty about what was the cause of these sudden ailments - food poisoning, gastric influenza and infant paralysis were all considered to be responsible for people's illness. Indeed news reports downplayed the seriousness of the epidemic and it was suggested that it was not so dangerous as previous examples. The *Birmingham Daily Post* claimed

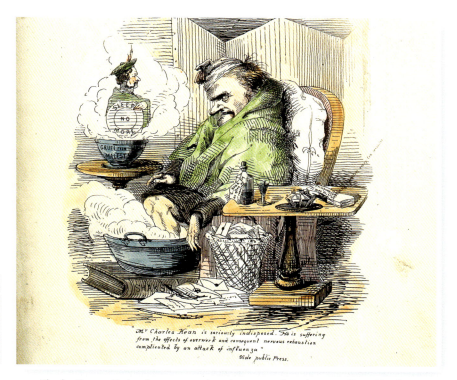

Charles Kean suffering from overwork and nervous exhaustion complicated by flu.

CHAPTER TWO

on 2 July that: 'Medical opinion is practically unanimous that the present epidemic is much milder than some previous visitations, for instance the epidemic of "Russian" influenza.' This view was shared by a writer in the *Staffordshire Advertiser* who suggested that fatalities were not from the flu but from complications, something that would be a common refrain in the months that followed.

For many of the population of the West Midlands the outbreak of influenza was intimately linked to the war and according to the *Birmingham Daily Post* in June 1918, 'the man in the street… is sometimes inclined to believe it is really a form of pro-German influence – the "unseen hand" is popularly supposed to be carrying test-tubes containing cultures of all the bacilli known to science, and many yet unknown'. These suspicions were not restricted to the region; in Washington State (USA) there were widely circulated reports that Lieutenant Phillip S. Doane, Head of the Health and Sanitation section of the Emergency Fleet Corporation had suggested German U-boats might have beached on their shores to spread the flu. A quarter of a million Germans died from disease. Nevertheless, for some who were hyper-patriotic the link between germs and Germans was very close and a number of nicknames emerged for the virus that embodied this prejudice, including: *Flanders Grippe, Hun flu, Turco-Germanic bacterial criminal enterprise*. Soldiers writing from the front or visiting Britain on leave or to convalesce also conveyed rumours that the heart of this 'German plague' lay in the unburied corpses on the battlefields or the Germans' use of poison gas.

Those who were not convinced that the influenza epidemic was the intentional work of the Axis powers often perceived it as an unintentional consequence of war and the arrival of groups of workers or troops from abroad. The French blamed the Spanish and in particular the Spanish workers who replaced French men who had joined the armed forces, whilst the Spanish singled out the Portuguese for blame. The Germans apparently suggested that the flu had been imported by the 100,000 men who worked behind the lines, assisting the Allies in France, as part of the Chinese Labour Corps. The sense that the conditions of war, the exhaustion, war weariness, the mixing of numerous strangers in the pursuit of the war, provided fertile ground for the spread of the disease had perhaps more credibility, but was again laced with a touch of anti-German feeling. Thus the *Birmingham Daily Post* argued on 25 June 1918:

CHAPTER TWO

> There can be no doubt whatever that it has been recurring in a very severe form in Germany, Austria, and the territories occupied by the Central Powers during the last two years. Malnutrition and the general weakening of nerve power known as war-weariness provide the necessary conditions for an epidemic, and contact between the national armies, which tends to make diseases international, is another factor favourable to propagation.

In 1918, there was no Ministry of Health to co-ordinate the gathering of information about influenza or to formulate policies. Public health was the responsibility of sanitary officers and local Medical Officers of Health – in Birmingham, Stafford and Worcester, for example. At a national level the Local Government Board had some responsibility for notifiable diseases but seems to have had a feeling of impotence regarding influenza – its Chief Medical Officer Sir Arthur Newsholme announced that he 'knew of no public health measures which can resist the progress of pandemic influenza'. Besides which, it was not really considered serious: after all, the vast majority of those who contracted the flu survived and were back at work within a few days. Not all were so lucky. Mr Allen Weaver, a 46-year-old slaughterman in Worcestershire, was taken ill one Thursday morning in early April 1918. He recovered during the day and towards the evening and apparently appeared almost himself; however, he died on the following Saturday evening. Faced with such sudden deaths, doctors struggled to understand the illness they were encountering. In part this was because they did not have the understanding of viruses which became common later in the twentieth century.

In 1918, bacteria had already been recognised as a cause of disease for decades, with specific species identified as the cause of individual diseases, including anthrax and cholera. Bacteria are generally easy to grow on petri dishes containing agar jelly, and specific staining conditions and shape of bacteria can give a good indication of the species. The prevailing wisdom of the time was that bacteria were responsible for influenza. A probable causative agent was identified by Richard Pfeiffer in 1892, and commonly known as Pfeiffer's bacillus. However, there was a problem with this theory. In order to prove the bacteria were responsible, they needed to be isolated from every case tested. This was not done: there were many cases from which the bacteria could

CHAPTER TWO

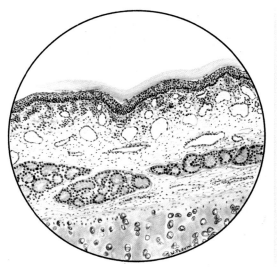

Drawing from 1918 by John George Adami of the trachea showing the earliest stage of reaction in influenza.

not be isolated. Around the same time, it was also becoming apparent, through work mostly on plants, that there was another type of disease-causing agent that was too small to be a bacterium, could not be grown on agar, but could be passed from host to host. These agents were named 'viruses' after the Latin word for poison although it was not clear what they actually were. It was not until the 1930s that work carried out on ferrets established that the true cause of influenza was a virus, thereafter called the influenza virus. The bacillus named after Richard Pfeiffer turned out to be the cause of a secondary infection, which can take hold in the affected lungs of influenza victims, causing further damage and increasing the chance of death. It is now known as *Haemophilus influenzae*, despite it having no relationship to the virus.

It was this widely held belief amongst doctors and scientists that flu was caused by bacteria that provided the backdrop for a plethora of advice on the importance of cleanliness and disinfectant from some newspaper journalists and medical professionals who even suggested gargling with disinfectant several times a day. Furthermore, the advertising industry drew upon these assumptions when they played upon people's fears and anxieties. Chymol First Aid Disinfectant Soap, for example, claimed that 'Flu has been conspicuous by its absence in homes' where the 'scientific disinfectant soap of guaranteed power' had been put into use. This magical soap was also apparently able to shake off influenza's ill-effects. One advert claimed 'Never since the Black Death has

CHAPTER TWO

INFLUENZA attacks the weak! Keep strong and well by taking Chymol

THE FOOD THAT BUILDS! (pronounced *KI-MOL*)

Doctors recommend Chymol both before and after Influenza.

Taken at once, Chymol will feed up your wartime weakened vitality, and increase your natural resistance to the prevalent germs.

If recovering from Influenza, Chymol will build up your strength and energy, quickly, and lastingly.

Its rich stores of red bone marrow, sweet fats, and fine Barley Malt are an endless source of strength to the healthiest or the weakest. Everybody needs Chymol today. All can digest it.

MADE IN ENGLAND

Chymol — The Food that Builds

1/4 & 2/10 at your Chemist or Stores.

Full particulars from THE CHYMOL CO., Ltd., Dept. 11E Queen's House, Kingsway, London, W.C.2.

Courtesy of the Library of Birmingham

Advert for one of a multitude of products sold to combat flu, *Birmingham Gazette*, 18 July 1918.

such a plague swept over the world as the recent epidemics of influenza… Influenza infection is by contact not airborne and this being so, it is certainly preventable.' It may have seemed a persuasive argument to the users of this and many other products who were not aware how the virus spread.

In the summer of 1918, winning the war was the priority at both national and local level. Thus concern about influenza in government circles focused on how it compromised the production of the vital machinery and supplies needed for war or the health of soldiers required for battle. A multitude of sources including newspapers, doctors, propaganda and politicians conveyed the message that in the face of a pandemic ordinary people should either ignore it, smile through the threat of illness or take care of themselves. The *Birmingham Mail* reassured its readers that 'fortunately the disease is not of a virulent type, carrying with it any actual danger'. Many in the Royal Army Medical Corps (RAMC) considered they had more pressing medical issues than flu, which was often seen in derisory terms as a mild complaint, compared to sepsis, gangrene, lice and enteric fevers. Whilst local newspapers did not receive the attention from the censors that national newspapers did, they all seemed to toe the government line and consider that the influenza was not generally something to write about in sensationalist terms.

It is now understood that a person with influenza is capable of spreading it to their family and friends for a day before symptoms appear, and for three to four days after they first appear. The virus normally replicates in the tissues of the nose and throat. It is now known to be spread by three different mechanisms: via liquid droplets released when people talk, cough or sneeze; as tiny airborne particles; and via contamination of solid objects, which are later touched by other people. The virus can remain active on these surfaces for hours, ready to infect the next person who touches them. The frequency with which each of these methods leads to infection is not entirely clear, and may vary in different environments, although it is thought that the droplet route is most significant as the virus can persist in the droplet for several hours and spread over a distance of up to six feet. Ultimately, using any of these methods, the virus has to get into the airways, and does so either by inhalation, or transmission from solid objects to the hands then to the face. Based on this modern understanding, the advice is to wash hands and surfaces regularly, and catch sneezes and coughs in disposable tissues.

Without this scientific knowledge, Spanish flu spread at some speed across the West Midlands. Concerns were increasingly expressed in local newspapers about how influenza interrupted everyday life and most importantly the war effort, causing schools to close and workforces to be depleted. German POWs who were needed to work on the land in the Evesham Vale were incapacitated by the flu. There were reports of flu in the army training camps on Cannock Chase. Courts struggled to function when witnesses or the police were too ill to attend and the *Birmingham Daily Mail* reported on 5 July that 'in one police division of the city nearly 30 constables failed yesterday to answer the roll call'. Likewise the carpet and spinning mills of Kidderminster were said to be 'suffering severely' as a result of the flu.

In the absence of any genuine scientific understanding of how the influenza actually spread and therefore how to get it under control, the local newspapers were full of different explanations and theories. Dirt, poor housing, the wartime propensity to dig up the land to grow more food, malnutrition, troops, and 'outsiders' were all held to be responsible for the spread of deadly flu virus. Even prior to the arrival of the flu, there was a sense that the movement of men in the armed forces dispersed diseases and epidemics across the country and between countries. The Headmaster of Coventry Street Boys' School in Kidderminster recorded in the school logbook on 7 February 1917 that 'scabies and other infectious complaints introduced by soldiers on leave (are) rather prevalent'.

During four years of conflict the battle against disease had often been as challenging as the battle against the enemy, of the 10 million military deaths that occurred across the world during the conflict, 3-4 million were from infectious diseases. These included tuberculosis, various forms of venereal disease and typhoid which was contracted from the lice that inhabited army uniforms. A vaccination had been developed for typhoid but as Worcestershire doctor Arthur Sladden, who had joined the Royal Army Medical Corps, explained to his father in a letter written on 14 October 1914, it was not uniformly welcomed:

Inoculation is voluntary and… it may produce considerable temporary illness. You can imagine that it is not always easy to persuade all the men to have it… Experience shows that inoculation reduces the incidence of disease 5 or 6 times and if inoculated people get it, their chances of recovery are much greater.

Against this background it is possible to understand the rumour that was circulating in Birmingham in the summer of 1918 suggesting that influenza was a version of trench fever, which had afflicted some 74,000 British troops. This also echoed the beliefs of many of

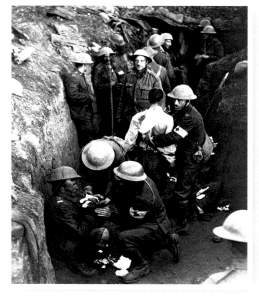

First World War regimental first aid post in the trenches. It was rumoured that death and disease at the front were responsible for causing influenza.

the medical profession who had trained in the 1880s before germ theory had developed, who still considered that diseases arose out of foetid conditions such as those to be found in the trenches. It was also linked to more general anxiety about troops, their experience of death and concerns that the death and disease of the battlefront would spread to the home front. Major E. C. Hawkshaw RA, who had seen active service in Ceylon, explained to the local newspapers in Worcester, under the heading *Fighting the so-called Influenza*:

> *There is in my mind, little doubt that the cause of it all is brought into the county by soldiers from our many fronts in the shape of microbes and insects saturated with putrid flesh and the unpleasant accompaniments inescapable from camps and battlefields. How then can this best be tackled?*
> *1) Keep cottages aired and clean; whitewash everywhere, if possible, and disinfect.*
> *2) If quinine runs short, drink tea made out of dandelion roots cut up and boiled, giving a small glassful daily to everyone in the house. Microbes dislike acids.*
> *3) Light a bonfire at odd times, near the house and let the smoke fumigate everything.*
> *4) As soon as a man returns from abroad (a) make him thoroughly wash himself all over, especially his hair (b) thoroughly disinfect his clothes and every single thing which he brings with him, omitting nothing. His whole kit is full of the eggs of these animals, all of which hatch out, as soon as he sits by the kitchen fire, thriving on any dust and dirt in the surroundings. Baking in the oven is a simple and good disinfectant.*
> *5) Keep Cheerful.*
> *If the above are adhered to "influenza" will like cholera and other virulent epidemics quickly disappear – the more so if done at the port of embarkation for home or disembarkation.*

The suggestion that 'keeping cheerful' was important and the use of the words 'so-called influenza' in the title of Major Hawkshaw's vociferous instructions in the local newspaper are indicative of the tendency to dismiss the flu as nothing too serious, a minor matter, something of a joke even at times.

CHAPTER TWO

However, as rumours and gossip continued to spread, the *Birmingham Daily Post* noted on 2 July that 'there had been 10 deaths in the previous week' and men and women had apparently 'collapsed at work and had to be sent home in ambulances'. In the following weeks some more alarmist approaches to the flu suggested that not only was the death rate from influenza rising but influenza was a contributory factor in many other deaths, particularly those which were being attributed to pneumonia and bronchitis. In discussing *Catarrh and Influenza*, the Medical Officer of Health in Birmingham noted that: 'These ailments cause a larger amount of loss of time and, either directly or indirectly, a larger number of deaths in Birmingham than any other group of diseases, mainly because they are so frequently the starting point of bronchitis and pneumonia.'

There were genuine problems in identifying and reporting occurrences and deaths from the pandemic. At the beginning of 1918, influenza was not a notifiable disease, despite the seriousness of the Russian flu in the 1890s. Reporting it was not compulsory, as it was not considered a public health risk in the way that tuberculosis, pneumonia, measles and whooping cough were. Indeed influenza was most often referred to, both in local medical officer reports and in the notices of death that appeared in local newspapers, in combination with other diseases such as pneumonia, catarrh or occasionally measles. The death of 23-year-old Lillian Basford, who undertook voluntary war-work entertaining wounded soldiers, was attributed to pneumonia following influenza in summer 1918.

The spread of the disease in the West Midlands, a region so important for wartime industrial production, was a national concern. *The Times* reported on 2 July that the epidemic had a 'great hold on the Midlands' and attributed this to influenza's apparent tendency to attack those 'generally engaged in indoor occupations'. The report went on to claim that 'persons engaged in outdoor occupations are practically immune'. As the crisis deepened, evidence emerged to challenge this assertion. In the interim several schools were closed in Birmingham due to the large number of teachers affected. 'Hundreds of men and women are away from the large works' and people were advised to avoid public transport and told: 'it would be beneficial… if persons who were at work in offices… were to walk home instead of riding in closed public vehicles'. Time did little to decrease the multitude of sometimes contradictory or perverse advice provided by Medical Officers, doctors, nurses and newspapers on the

CHAPTER TWO

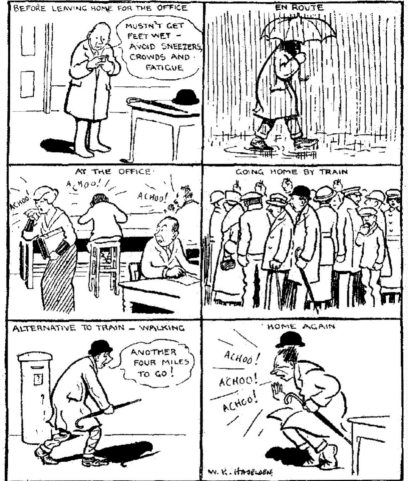

'How to Avoid Influenza' by W K Haselden, *Daily Mirror*, 25 October 1918.

appropriate actions to prevent, cure or aid recovery from the flu, including: fresh air, eating well, consuming large quantities of meat or to 'keep cheerful and laugh as much as you like' and even the organisation of sneezing parties. The Chymol Company suggested that worry, failure to digest food properly and lack of vitality were making people vulnerable to the disease and germs. The answer apparently lay in the consumption of their patent powder consumed in milk three times a day.

CHAPTER TWO

Despite the purchase of patent medicines, the pandemic continued to threaten productivity. The *Birmingham Daily Post* reported on 5 July that vital war work was in jeopardy: 'the output of some of the munitions factories is badly affected, girls being the principal patients'. In London Sir Arthur Newsholme, the Chief Medical Officer of the Local Government Board drew up plans to cut absenteeism in munitions factories by providing extra nursing staff, or staggering working hours, but they were not acted upon: he was concerned they might cause panic and the priority above all else was the war effort. Munitions factories in the Black Country instead relaxed their no smoking rules as smoke was deemed able to prevent the spread of the illness. It was also suggested that gas prevented the spread of flu and that gas workers had lower mortality rates. Alternatively, miners genuinely had a higher rate of mortality, something that has been linked to the weakened state of miners' lungs due to inhaling mineral dusts. In Staffordshire, determined miners, who brought up the coal needed to power factories and ships, continued to work even when not fully recovered from the influenza. According to the *Walsall Observer and South Staffordshire Chronicle*, this led to a number of deaths from pneumonia in Cannock Chase in July. In the month that followed there continued to be concern that the output of coal was being checked by the number of miners absent from work as a consequence of influenza in the region; this time the problem was most acute in Burntwood.

Dr Robertson, the Medical Officer of Health, explained to the Birmingham Public Health Committee in the middle of July that '69 deaths last week were due to influenza' but then went on to suggest that 'it was probably more correct to say 140-150 deaths were due directly to the malady'. The different fatality figures are indicative of the awareness of how difficult many doctors found diagnosis in this era based upon external examination of the patient on death. There was neither the time, money nor the inclination for post-mortems to be undertaken, something which families also regarded as anathema. He continued his report by saying that he believed that 'the worst of the outbreak had passed'. This was to be a constant refrain amongst both medical experts and journalists in the region throughout the pandemic. Nationally, the influenza epidemic was reported to have abated by the middle of August, but not before it had killed 130 people in Stoke-on-Trent in July and August alone.

CHAPTER TWO

As the summer of 1918 drew to a close and the news not only from the Western Front but also from those fighting in Palestine was positive, hope began to grow for the residents of the West Midlands that the end of the conflict and the carnage was in sight. Likewise families began to hope that the end of 1918 would bring if not celebration, then at least relief. Fate, however, dealt a cruel blow. A wet, cold and windy September heralded the second wave of influenza that struck the region in October 1918. Although initially it was thought that the autumn attack was not so virulent as the previous wave, in fact it proved to be more deadly. As Dr Robertson, the Medical Officer of Health in Birmingham explained: 'No epidemic of influenza in previous times was so extensive in its prevalence.'

CHAPTER THREE

The enemy on the home front

In October 1918, as the nation turned its focus to the final stages of the war, a new more deadly version of the Spanish flu was spreading through the population of the West Midlands and their relatives on the Western Front. Nevertheless, the Medical Officer of Health in Worcester continued to maintain that combating this disease was 'purely a personal matter' and that the spread was 'due to the carelessness of individuals'. The *Worcester Daily Times* on 23 October 1918 issued the following instructions to residents of the area, which again relying on the assumptions that flu was a bacterial rather than a viral disease:

> Constantly flush pea rooms [toilets] and living rooms with fresh air. Avoid overcrowded rooms and places of amusement. Not more than one person to one room for sleeping purposes where anyone is affected. The wet cleansing of all infected places is important. Indiscriminate spitting is especially dangerous. Prolonged mental strain or over-fatigue, and still more alcoholism, should be avoided. The only safe rule is to regard all catarrhal attacks and every illness associated with rise in temperature as infectious and to adopt at once precautionary measures… Sneezing and coughing in public should be avoided where possible and in every case a handkerchief should be held in front of the face.

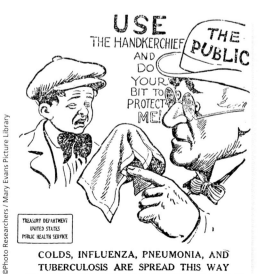

An image created by the famous cartoonists, Clifford T. Berryman in 1918 to educate the population.

CHAPTER THREE

The living conditions, crowded housing and fatigue which this advice suggested should be avoided were a way of life to many working class families in the region. The *Worcester Daily Times* reported how the head of a family and another member of the same family had lain in bed ill with flu in two rooms, whilst a child lay dead in another. Furthermore, many like Mabel Victoria Turner, whose demise was discussed in the *Worcester Daily Times* on 18 October 1918, lived in crowded lodging houses. One Monday early in October, she complained of a cough and the following day went to see the doctor who diagnosed her as suffering from influenza, gave her a prescription and sent her home to bed. Witnesses suggested that although Mabel returned home she did not go to bed or at least did not stay there. On Wednesday morning she came downstairs in the lodging house where she lived at 2 Little Boughton Street, Worcester and after obtaining a drink returned to bed for the day. A young mother who resided in the same house came downstairs to get medicine for her small son at 6:30 on Thursday morning. As she passed Mabel's door, she observed her sitting on her bed with her head thrown back, dead. According to her fellow residents in the lodging house Mabel, despite being only 21 years old, had previously suffered from poor health and difficulty breathing and 'had fits'. The doctor's post-mortem indicated she had had pleurisy and pneumonia in the past, but the doctor's view, accepted by the coroner, was that Mabel died of heart failure due to acute influenza.

Given the ambiguity of some medical diagnosis and advice it was perhaps not surprising that journalists, local or national politicians and the chattering classes continued to seek to explain the spread of the influenza. In the late nineteenth and early twentieth century there was a justifiable sense that it was healthier to live in rural areas than industrial cities; this may have led to both under- and over-reporting of illness and death as a result of the pandemic. In Birmingham influenza was considered to be severe whilst rural Hereford claimed to be almost untouched. The much greater density of population in Birmingham would have facilitated the spread of the flu, but it was dirt, poverty and a lack of clean air which were blamed.

The association of influenza with areas of poverty and people who were under-nourished was not, however, supported by individual reports of deaths, nor did it correlate with the many areas to which the illness had spread. Indeed the Spanish flu was a remarkably democratic illness, affecting the wealthy and the privileged as frequently as the poor. In the village Belbroughton, according to the *Berrow's Worcester Journal* on 18 October 1918: 'This scourge has laid its hold on the district and several fatal cases have occurred from it, or its sequel pneumonia. Mr Harbach of Bourne Castle, Mr Crips of Fairfield and Mrs F.A. Whatmore of this village succumbed after surprisingly short illnesses. Only two weeks later it was reported that in Martley Edith Margaret Nash, the daughter of Mr and Mrs Slade Nash, was a victim of the influenza epidemic. She belonged to a highly respected family who had lost two sons in the war.'

Likewise, the Duke of Orleans, the great-grandson of Louis Phillippe, the last King of France who maintained a residence at Wood Norton Hall, near Evesham in Worcestershire contracted and survived the flu in October 1918. Fatalities were not restricted to the poor living in lodging houses or to those who could not afford good food, but also included the well-off middle classes. Mr J. G. Nicol, a glove manufacturer of 26 years, also died of flu. He had worked as a manager for Dent, Allcroft and Co. and then established his own factory in New Street and St Martin's Gate, Worcester and was famous for using those parts of leather which were not suitable for gloves to make gaiters, purses and braces. Local newspapers carried reports of the rich and famous who died in this second wave of influenza: these included Sir Hubert Parry, composer of the coronation music for King George V, as well as the eldest son of the author, Sir Arthur Conan Doyle.

Furthermore, rural areas, particularly ones like the fruit and vegetable growing areas of Evesham Vale in Worcestershire, with 14 railway stations and a steady influx of people to work on farms, stay in convalescence hospitals or enjoy a day trip were badly affected by influenza. Consequently, farmers and market gardeners, even though they worked outdoors did not escape the flu or its potentially fatal consequences. In Badsey in the Evesham Vale, Mr Fred Stewart's family of 11 were all suffering from flu in late October. Indeed the whole village of Badsey, with its POW camp containing over 200 Germans who were working on the land, was considered to be one of the worst areas in the region for the influenza. Both prisoners and their guards caught the virus.

Nearby Mr Henry Smith Rimell, a 55-year-old farmer with considerable experience of managing farms in the district and 700 acres under his control in the village of Bishampton died within a week of contracting influenza, despite being considered to be a fit and healthy man. He apparently excelled at growing

CHAPTER THREE

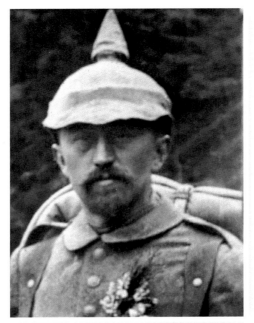

Johann Rosskopf, POW in Badsey, Worcestershire, who died of influenza on 14 November 1918.

the corn that was so important for making bread to feed the population in wartime. He was a pillar of the rural community, sitting on the Evesham Horse Show Committee and the Pershore Board of Guardians, as well as being a Church Warden and an official with the National Farmers Union. Hence his funeral was well attended; but not by two of his daughters who were themselves suffering from influenza.

In some of the conjecture about influenza there was, problematically, both anxiety and condemnation of working class culture and ways of life that had developed in response to economic hardship and uncertainty. The *Bromsgrove, Droitwich and Redditch Weekly Messenger* considered that 'fatigue, exposure, want of nourishing food and intemperance all make people more susceptible' and went on to link influenza to wartime food shortages. In the first half of the twentieth century, there was a tendency to assume that lack of education, laziness or the obtuseness of working class housewives were responsible for the poor nutrition of the working classes. There has been some debate since amongst historians about whether the standard of health and nutrition of the wartime population improved or deteriorated during the conflict. Investigations carried out at the time and since suggest that during wartime there was an overall reduction in the consumption of sugar, cheese, butter, butcher's meat, fruit and vegetables, whilst more bacon, sausages, and margarine were eaten. There was also apparently a reduction in the consumption of certain vitamins such as A and B12, C, D, and riboflavin which may have had a detrimental effect on some people's general health. However, this does not explain the spread or severity of an influenza pandemic, which was by no means concentrated on the geographical areas or social classes with the poorest diets.

Concern about working class drinking had been a preoccupation for middle class temperance reformers since the nineteenth century. They had had some success as the opening hours of public houses and the strength of the beer had been cut during the conflict, in the hope this would improve wartime manufacturing productivity. Some temperance reformers clearly envisaged that the influenza pandemic could be utilised to serve their cause. Others continued to suggest that poverty and poor living conditions were responsible for the spread of influenza or for the failure to recover from the illness. As the *Worcester Daily Times* proposed:

The lowered vitality of our people owing to the tremendous worry, the food conditions and the coal conditions was certainty one cause of the epidemic Another main cause was the crowding together of men of all classes and from all parts of the world and on transports.

The debate about causation continued in the local press and an alternative view was put forward in the *Evesham Journal*, which pointed out on 2 November that: 'All classes of the community are affected, and it appears to take an even more virulent form with the apparently hale and hearty.' Villages, it was reported, were 'suffering equally badly' and numerous deaths in rural areas had occurred.

The local newspaper reports both of coroners' investigations and of the verdicts they reached regarding causes of death suggest doctors diagnosing influenza were also struggling with uncertainty. At times they seem to have been hunting to identify external factors, which could explain why one person died and another survived. Some, like Mabel Turner, were suggested to be in poor health prior to contracting flu and any complications such as pneumonia were attributed to this. In other cases it was the suddenness of the death of a person previously seen to be in robust health which seems to be an important factor in doctors suggesting a diagnosis of flu. When Lillian Queenie Gilbert, aged 19 months, died one morning asleep in her bed in Worcestershire, the doctor, who seems to have found no visible signs or symptoms, attributed the death to influenza, as the child was clean and well nourished. The mother's explanation that the child had been delicate from birth was ignored. The tendency to attribute any unexplained death to influenza raises questions about some of the figures for mortality rates. Occasionally there was an admission of this uncertainty as when the *Worcester Daily Times* newspaper reported on the demise of Edith Eileen Knight – under the heading *Influenza Suspected* at the end of October 1918. Edith was the wife of Charles Knight, a carpet weaver in Stourport, who had been in good health until she had gone to bed suffering from a cold. Early the following day she had stomach pains and asked for a cup of cocoa but as she was looking very ill, a neighbour advised that the doctor should be sent for, but Edith died before he arrived.

In the middle of October, the Medical Officer of Health for Worcester, Mabyn Read, was quoted in the local newspaper, stating that 'the influenza that was now raging in the city is widespread and severe'. Fifteen deaths from influenza were reported the previous week in the city. The newspapers described the 'scourge' of flu as so prevalent 'that it might almost rank with a plague in long past days'. By the beginning of November the local press in Worcester carried reports, not only of six people dying in one day in Worcester but also of there having been 7,417 deaths in England and Wales the previous week, up from 4,482 the week before. Likewise there were reports that the disease was still widespread in Evesham and Stourport. Over 1,500 cases were reported in Kidderminster, which was considered to be particularly badly hit, with carpet and spinning mills again suffering severely from absenteeism.

For many people in the region, the influenza was seen as yet another hardship brought about by war, and the disease added to the general depression and malaise for the war weary population. In Stoke-on-Trent there were 64 deaths from the pandemic in the week leading up to 26 October. Yet in Birmingham there was still a reticence, even as the numbers of fatalities climbed, to recognise the seriousness of this new wave of influenza. Although some factories and businesses were once again complaining that they were suffering from depleted staff due to illness and absenteeism, two other factories responded

Adverts such as this mistakenly suggested that disinfectant could combat the spread of the flu. *Birmingham Post*, 6 November 1918.

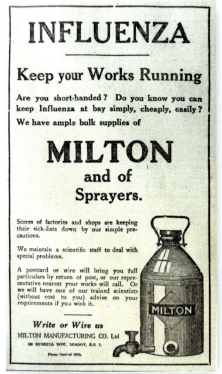

to an inquiry from the *Birmingham Daily News* by stating that influenza was spreading but not at such an alarming rate as previously and they only had about 100 cases, whereas in the summer they had witnessed between 3,000 and 4,000 cases. Some factories looked for preventative measures to stop the spread of flu. Advertisements sought to address the need to keep manufacturing works running; it was, for example, suggested that by spraying their premises with Milton disinfectant, employers could avoid factories or offices becoming short-staffed through sickness. To facilitate such industrial-scale use, the product could be ordered in bulk.

Some people were, however, beginning to comprehend the seriousness of the situation and becoming increasingly worried; these sought to take action to prevent the spread of influenza. An officer commanding troops in the region announced in the *Birmingham Daily Mail* on 30 October that owing to the influenza epidemic all theatres, music halls, picture houses and places of entertainment had been placed out of bounds for troops, hospital staff and patients in Birmingham and the counties of Warwick and Worcester. The region's vital war work had contributed to a sense of regional identity and pride but during the pandemic this seems to have clouded judgements and officials were keen to downplay the number of deaths in their areas compared to others. Consequently, despite the news of 95 deaths from influenza the previous week in the city, the *Birmingham Gazette* in early November continued to try and reassure the population that the city was not as badly affected as some others.

CHAPTER THREE

This must have been of little comfort to those living with family tragedies caused by influenza. There were reports of many houses where two members of the family were lying dead, or whole families were ill with the virus. In one family in Selly Oak, the husband, wife and daughter all died of influenza within a fortnight of one another. Finally, as the month progressed, and the war drew to an end, it became increasingly clear that the death toll from flu in the city was rising alarmingly and Birmingham's pride in not being as afflicted by the flu as other towns was misplaced.

The news of an armistice on Monday 11 November was celebrated with a torchlight procession in Malvern, Worcestershire. This involved hundreds of Boy Scouts, the band of the Church Lads' Brigade, Girl Guides, wounded soldiers and young women in fancy-dress costumes, an effigy of Britannia in a chariot, and a model of the Kaiser in a wicker chair, which was later placed on a bonfire around which there was dancing. In Tunstall, Staffordshire, Edith Birchall noted that 'the market square thronged with men, women and children who did no more work that day'. Crowds likewise packed the main streets of Birmingham on Monday and Tuesday evening. Undergraduates from the university, munitions

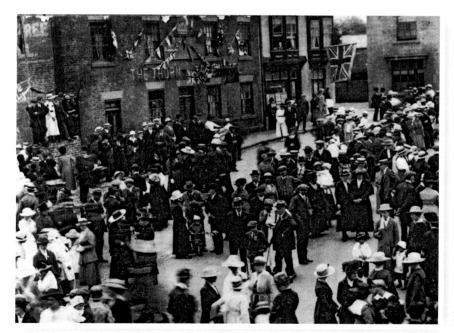

Celebrating the end of the Fir World War, Market Place, Ripley, Derbyshire (1918). Armistice day celebrations like this one helped spread the deadly virus.

CHAPTER THREE

workers, members of the Women's Army Auxiliary Corps and land girls all fraternised with each other. Amidst the song and dance policemen were embraced by the crowds. Descriptions can found for similar celebrations and revelry all across the West Midlands. All such celebrations provided an ideal opportunity for the influenza virus to be passed from one person to another. Even the famous Birmingham Chamberlain family was not immune. Ida Chamberlain wrote from rural Hampshire to her brother Neville at her regret at not being in the thick of the peace celebrations:

> *I must say I felt I should have liked to be in London or some place where one could meet one's fellow man en masse but perhaps Beatrice at any rate does not seem to have benefitted much from being on the spot; spending her day at some committees & ladies meeting in the evening.*

Beatrice, her sister went on to note, had apparently caught 'the flu into the bargain'. A keen participant on a number of committees in London covering areas such as the British Red Cross, Food Economy and War Savings, Beatrice was very active in the Children's Country Holidays Fund for Fulham and Kensington, and died of the influenza on 19 November 1918.

November saw influenza begin to wane in many areas of Britain but as historian Niall Johnson points out, in the week ending 16 November, parts of the Midlands, Wales, Yorkshire and the northeast were showing an increase in mortality from the disease. Kidderminster had its worst week of the pandemic in mid-November but in Worcester Dr Mabyn Read, the Medical Officer of Health, continued to reassure the local population that although there had been 41 deaths from flu in the city the previous week the 'disease is past its worst'. This was one example of many, as across the region officials and newspapers continued to try and bolster public morale with this oft-repeated mantra. Increasing numbers of people were encountering the deadly virus amongst their family or friends, so these exhortations were wearing very thin. In Birmingham the funeral took place of a family of four who lived in rented accommodation in William Street, Lozells and had all died within hours of each other from influenza. They were buried in one grave at Witton Cemetery.

If in April 1918 there had been much encouragement to stoically carry on

CHAPTER THREE

for the sake of the war effort, this approach was abandoned in the last days of the conflict and in the months after its conclusion. National newspapers lost their reticence about discussing the severity of the crisis, for which they received some criticism. Hilda Chamberlain writing to her brother Neville, the future Birmingham Ladywood MP and later Prime Minister, claimed that the coverage of the *Influenza Scare* in *The Times* was 'about as low as anything *The Times* has done up to now'. To her the fuss being made about influenza was all political manoeuvring by those seeking to carve out roles for themselves in new government departments around health. Newspapers now openly likened the epidemic to Russian Flu of the 1890s but also more alarmingly to the Black Death, sweating sickness and other plagues of the Tudor era. There were stories of the horrors of influenza from towns and cities in Britain and across the world, for example. in Petrograd and Odessa, Pretoria and Cape Town. That influenza was an international pandemic, something with a reach well beyond the countries involved in fighting on the Western Front, was beginning to dawn on people, increasing their sense of panic and unease.

Local newspapers also propagated urban myths of the grizzly impact of the disease, based upon hearsay from other parts of the country. For example, they reported the example of 'a rather foreign looking man, the head packer at the co-operative store in Stowmarket' who had apparently beaten his wife and children to death before hanging himself as a consequence of melancholy brought on by the flu. In popular culture, the Russian Flu epidemic had been associated with patients being left with a long period of melancholy and depression. There were fears that this new pandemic would have the same consequences, something to which the case of Lily Green from West Bromwich seemed to give credibility. She had been suffering with influenza at home in King Street, where she lived with her husband. But she went missing and apparently 'her body, clad only in her nightdress, was found in the Birmingham canal'.

As the wartime restrictions on censorship began to loosen, the full scale of the crisis became clearer in the West Midlands where there was no let up to the illness or the death it brought. On 21 November 1918 the *Birmingham Evening Dispatch* noted that unlike other areas, the death rate in Birmingham, Coventry, Nottingham, Manchester and Bradford had increased the previous week. Under the headline *Birmingham one of the towns where malady is worse* the following figures for deaths for the previous week were given:

CHAPTER THREE

Newspaper reports of deaths in one week in November 1918 population

West Ham	161
Birmingham	246
Nottingham	198
Bradford	122
Sheffield	241
Coventry	110
Manchester	235
Leeds	208
Dublin	141
Bristol	144

When Dr Robertson, the Medical Officer of Health in Birmingham, came to write his report for 1918, he carefully charted the deaths from influenza in the city. Even accepting the inaccuracy that may have surrounded figures that relied upon coroners' findings rather than detailed medical reports, the sharp rise in deaths caused by the pandemic from the middle of October to the middle of December could not be ignored. It reached a peak in late November with more than 300 deaths in the city within a week. As he explained when discussing flu more generally:

> *The average number of deaths from this disease during each of the years 1913-1917 was 129. During 1918 there were 2,172 deaths directly attributable to it. There was, in addition, an excessive mortality from Pneumonia of 256 deaths, about the average, and it is safe to say that the disease was directly or indirectly the cause of at least 2,500 deaths. That is, one out of every five deaths, which occurred during the year, was due to influenza.*

The consequences of these figures for doctors, undertakers and everyday life will be explored in later chapters but it is also important to remember that anxiety about influenza in the West Midlands did not just focus on those on the home front. Many had loved ones in the forces who, as the risk from enemy fire

CHAPTER THREE

was eliminated, were still vulnerable to the influenza virus which swept through army and POW camps abroad.

Influenza ensured that the armistice did not bring an end to the death toll among young people, nor did the armistice bring a speedy return of men in the fighting forces to their loved ones. For those on the home front at the end of 1918, life was overshadowed by anxiety about when and whether their husbands, brothers, fathers or sweethearts would return from arenas of battle or POW camps abroad. There was a terrible fear that influenza would at the last moment snatch away the future that they had longed for during several years of war. Throughout the autumn news had reached the Midlands of men in the forces dying, not from their injuries but from influenza and its complications. Bromsgrove soldier Thomas Wallace had been a driver delivering milk prior to joining up in October 1914, aged only 17. He served in France from 1915, only to die in a casualty clearing station of pneumonia which had developed from influenza, on 10 November 1918 at the age of just 21.

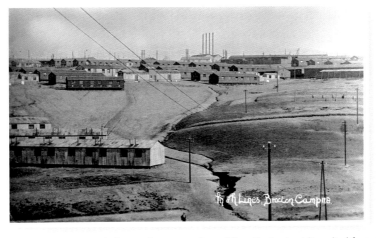

Brocton camp on Cannock Chase where a number of New Zealand soldiers died from flu.

Thousands of soldiers of the New Zealand Rifle Brigade had been stationed at Brocton Military Camp on Cannock Chase in Staffordshire, training to take part in hostilities in Europe. By the end of 1918, 40 of them had been buried in the cemetery there, unable to return home, victims of the influenza. They were not alone in having avoided the horror and danger of the trenches only to succumb to the disease. Bombardier E.C.G. Vale from

CHAPTER THREE

Bromsgrove had worked for 10 years in the office at the Royal Enfield Cycle Company prior to the conflict. He joined up under the Derby Scheme in 1916, and was expected home on leave to get married in December 1918. He, like the New Zealand riflemen, never returned, having died of influenza.

There was also bad news for many young wives whose soldier-husbands died of influenza in POW camps abroad before they could be repatriated. Jack Marsh of Dudley in the Black Country had volunteered in 1914 and had endured four years of war but by autumn 1918 was in a POW camp in Turkey, from where he wrote to his brother on 8 October to say that 'he was all right'. He also mentioned that 'the Spanish influenza was very prevalent' in the camp, and eight days after the armistice, aged only 26, he died of influenza. As his brother told the local newspapers, this 'makes the sorrow and regret double, for it was within the bounds of possibility that he would soon be home again'.

The popular wartime song 'Good-bye-ee', written and composed in 1917, was rewritten to address the threat of influenza with the words:

Don't cry-ee, don't sigh-ee,
There's a silver lining in the sky-ee
Bonsoir old thing, cheerio, chin-chin,
Nah-poo, take the flu and die-ee

The anxieties that were experienced by many soldiers are conveyed in a letter from Cyril Cartwright, stationed in France, to his wife at home in Birmingham as he waited to be released from the armed forces in December 1918.

Well Gerties we are still here with no news of moving at present and no signs of coming home either so we have to be content with the present position...

Flu I believe is very bad again at home so you must be extra careful. We are rather depressed at the company at present one of own officers has just died from the flu and what makes the case harder he was a 1914 man and is married so you see how hard it is and that is why I keep impressing upon you to be most careful. I feel pretty well myself except a

CHAPTER THREE

little bit of a cold which I usually get, every thing is quite alright and I am looking after myself as well as I possibly can so please don't worry about me too much.

Cyril's awareness of the danger of influenza on the home front and in army camps would also have been intensified by news of comrades whose wives were ill or had died. Hugo Fidoe from Worcestershire had been a prisoner of war in Turkey since Easter Sunday in 1916, and his wife died of flu on the day of the armistice. Another soldier was recalled from the army to be at the bedside of his wife and two young children, struck down by influenza. After his return to his regiment, his wife lost her battle with the illness and died whilst his children remained poorly. One Birmingham resident recently recounted that they had:

read a letter from my great-grandmother to her husband posted in India, she wrote it just a few weeks before the flu took her; she wrote that she was beginning to think that she would never get her voice back properly again and that she was not feeling very well, she wrote that she thought she might try and get a dispensary note.

When she died her husband was away in India and a telegram was sent to call him back, we have the faded copy still.

Her mother had to look after the children… they all lived in back to backs in Benacre Street in Balsall Heath.

Some men in the forces, like Lance Corporal John Henry Turner from Stoke-on-Trent, found that their war was prematurely cut short by influenza, but few kept a diary charting their experience of the flu as he did. John was on active service with the Signal Company of the Royal Engineers in Northern France in October 1918 when he was taken ill. On reporting to the doctor, he was told he had a chill and given some pills. However, the next morning he was unable to get up and realised that he 'was indeed very ill'. The doctors were all too busy, no doubt struggling with the consequences of the Spanish flu, and he lay all day without attention. In the morning, John got up and went to find a doctor, struggling not to faint while waiting his turn. When the doctor examined

CHAPTER THREE

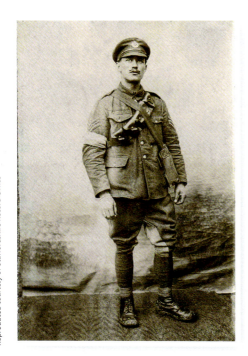

John Henry Turner whose war was cut short when he contracted flu.

him, the seriousness of John's illness was realised and he was transferred in an ambulance to the 5th Casualty Clearing Station at Corbie where he was ordered to bed with a high temperature. For the next five nights John was cared for by the medical staff, including a sister he described as 'kindness itself'. On 4 November he was wrapped up in blankets and a pneumonia jacket. This medical device was made of oiled silk, muslin and occasionally incorporated rubber tubes that could circulate hot water, all with the intention of keeping patients warm.

To his surprise John was ordered back to Britain and was transported via hospital train to Le Havre, before crossing the Channel by hospital ship to Southampton, and thence by hospital train and stretcher to Eden Hall Voluntary Aid Detachment (VAD) hospital, Edenbridge, Kent where he was put to bed straight away. On visiting the next morning the doctor instructed the nurse to get him a hot water bottle; however, it was midday before it arrived. When he was told he could get up for a bit, after he had been up for about an hour, he found he was struggling for breath. He had developed pneumonia, and later recalled in his diary that he would never forget the experience, as he suffered. for days.

Unwilling to allow the hospital to contact his wife and as he was, like most in this era, a religious man, he put his faith in 'the Lord' to see him through. Advisable perhaps as he seems to have been underwhelmed by the VADs who worked in the hospital and who he considered were more concerned with drinking tea with the doctors than with re-filling his hot water bottle. Nevertheless, because of or despite the nursing care he received, he made

CHAPTER THREE

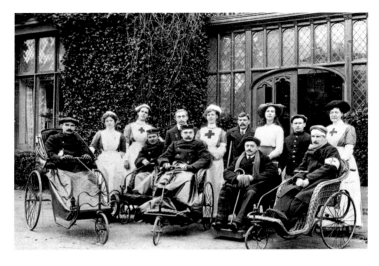

Eden Hall VAD Hospital, Edenbridge, Kent, Christmas Day 1914, where four years later John Henry Turner recovered from flu caught while serving in France.

progress towards recovery and later recorded: 'Well I did mend eventually and I knew it when I was being given Roast Chicken, my dearest wish was I could have it with my wife.'

As his health slowly improved, he asked the doctor if he could go home; however, on discovering that John's home was in the Potteries, this member of the medical profession noted this was 'not exactly a health resort'. Nevertheless John was given 10 days' hospital-leave to recuperate in domestic surroundings and by the time he was fully recovered the conflict was over. He and his wife could breathe a sigh of relief that he had survived both enemy fire and influenza; they could start to rebuild their lives together in Stoke-on-Trent. The influenza epidemic itself subsided at the end of December 1918, allowing the West Midlands to breathe a collective sigh of relief. For some areas, the end of this wave largely meant the end of the flu epidemic altogether, according to George Newman's *Report on the Pandemic of Influenza 1918-9* for the first Minister of Health, Christopher Addison. For other areas, a third wave of flu was on its way in 1919.

CHAPTER FOUR

Bovril and whisky: everyday life during the influenza pandemic

It has been estimated that approximately ten million people in Britain contracted influenza between 1918 and 1919, of whom 2.5% or 228,000 individuals died. There were still many, many more people who caught the virus but did not die, as the *Worcester Daily Times* explained on 4 November 1918. 'There have been a large number of cases where, no complications having arisen, the patients have been able to get about after a few days.' Details of the lives of those who died can be found in the notices of their death that appeared in the newspapers along with reports from coroners' courts, but it is harder to find evidence of how influenza was experienced in everyday life for those who contracted the illness and recovered. They sought remedies, worried what would be the outcome of the influenza for them and dealt with the aftermath of the virus but left only traces of their encounters with influenza in newspapers, diaries and oral histories.

In June 1918, a journalist described his experiences of the flu for an advertising feature in the *Birmingham Daily Post*. His account was shaped perhaps by the financial incentive he may have received from the manufacturer of a medicine that claimed would help cure the influenza, but it provides a vivid narrative. According to this journalist, the symptoms of flu included 'a swift loss of mental capacity, an inability to think coherently' which he 'found most distressing'. However, as soon as he knew his temperature was too high, he apparently took the 'prescription of the De Goncourt brothers for all the ills of life, from an unfavourable criticism to an excess of world sorrow' and went to bed in company with a hot-water bottle. He claimed that bed and quinine were the best preventatives of complications from the disease and expressed the view that it was struggling against or ignoring influenza that led to bronchitis or pneumonia. Like many in the first wave of the pandemic, whilst the First World War was still raging, he played down the seriousness of influenza and its after-effects. He considered these were much less debilitating, in the long term, than his memory of catching Russian flu in the 1890s, which had left him suffering from melancholy for many months. Others were less convinced that the after-

CHAPTER FOUR

effects were so quickly thrown off, as evidenced by the numerous adverts from the hair specialist J. Green recommending his tonic to restore hair after influenza in many West Midlands newspapers.

The *Birmingham Daily Post* journalist was not alone. Descriptions of the experience of suffering from influenza and accompanying endorsements for particular products filled the pages of local newspapers. Miss Heywood apparently found herself in a very low state of health, from which she thought she was never going to recover, after suffering a bout of influenza. Her long-term symptoms, she claimed, included headaches and fainting attacks as 'the dregs of the flu seemed to have mastered' her. The answer to her problems lay in *Dr Williams' Pills for Pale People*, which indeed contained ferrous sulphate and would have been a helpful antidote to anaemia, but were pricier and weaker than

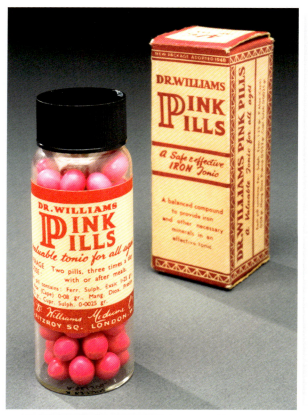

Dr Williams' 'Pink Pills', London, England, 1850-1920, sold to the desperate public to alleviate the symptoms of flu.

the iron tablets that were available from doctors. They were an international brand, which had been on sale since the middle of the nineteenth century and were apparently a cure for all manner of complaints, including pulmonary tuberculosis, rheumatism, paralysis, heart disease, rickets, dyspepsia, eczema, St. Vitus' dance and menstrual disorders as well as influenza. Many who displayed symptoms indicating they had caught the flu were anxious and willing to spend money trying to increase their chances of survival and importantly to prevent influenza from developing into something more serious. This was an era in which many of the population, sometimes unwilling or unable to pay for a doctor, resorted to patent medicines. The pandemic opened up a plethora of opportunities for charlatans and spurious claims from manufacturers that their products would prevent, cure or help recovery from the flu. Dr Williams' Pills were advertised as helping to counter the 'after-effects of the influenza and build up the blood'. Testimonials suggested not only that many remained in rude health due to the regular consumption of the little tablets but also that those who had grown weak from the flu gained colour and appetite and were able to eat again and grew in strength after regularly taking the tablets.

Those who had not experienced influenza directly within their family were all too aware it was sweeping through the region. Families like that of Elizabeth Cross who lived in Birmingham who later recalled:

> *it was terrible … everyone you spoke to had got relations, people down with influenza and we didn't. We were lucky really I think, you know, it affected a lot of people what was under nourished and people like that you know, yes there was oh such a lot of people died with that. I remember that just vaguely in a child way you know it's a funny thing, things like that doesn't affect your family and you're young. You don't seem to remember it so much, you know.*

Elizabeth would have been aware of the influenza epidemic not just because of individuals whose families were decimated but because of the attempts by the Medical Officers of Health to restrict the spread of the disease – particularly during the most lethal second wave between October and December 1918. In all likelihood her school would have been closed at least for a while but the overwhelming sense of panic influenza engendered led to what

CHAPTER FOUR

were, in retrospect, perhaps some useful restrictions introduced around public gatherings held in music halls and theatres and at football matches.

Some of the decisions about which mass events or activities were curtailed arguably owed a lot to already existing prejudices about working class culture and entertainment. For example, there seems to be no evidence of anyone trying to discourage church services although many people mingled together for worship. Cinema and football were a particular focus for control, with soldiers often prevented from entering football grounds, to avoid them both catching and spreading the deadly virus. In early November, soldiers were refused admission to an afternoon football match between Birmingham City and Hull City. The management stated that they were following orders from military authorities but there was much disappointment as it had been thought that it was unventilated buildings which were the focus of concern, not people standing together in the open air. Once again the debate about what should or should not be done was shaped by the misapprehension that influenza was a bacteria not an airborne virus.

As a relatively new and working class entertainment, cinema had first begun to gain popularity in the early 1900s, although the mass of the population gathered together in the dark had caused some disquiet. In the early days of cinema, the audience was occasionally sprayed with disinfectant to prevent the spread of disease. The terms of their licence meant that proprietors of cinemas and theatres could be compelled, under certain circumstances, to exclude children of school age, and to provide intervals for the efficient ventilation of the building. During the pandemic, the licences were interpreted locally and cinemas across the region became the focus of all sorts of regulations about ventilation, the disinfecting of their drapes and other cleanliness measures. Cinemas in Wolverhampton were ordered to ban children and remove all carpets. The Worcester Medical Officer's Report considered that the decisions to prevent children under 14 from entering the cinema and ensure that there was plenty of ventilation between performances were important factors in counteracting the spread of influenza. In many areas the practice of continuous performances was modified, so that in Wolverhampton for example, an interval was created between 5:00 and 6:30 each evening. Likewise a 60-minute interval was placed in the middle of Saturday morning children's showings in some areas, also to permit thorough ventilation of the building.

CHAPTER FOUR

> **'FLU AND THE CINEMA.**
>
> Effect of the New Order in Birmingham.
>
> **Bombshell for Cinemas.**
>
> The drastic regulation known as "The Influenza Order," issued yesterday was a bombshell to many members of the entertainment industry. The Order stipulates that there shall be no performance of more than three hours' duration and that a period of something like 30 minutes shall be allowed between each performance in order that in the interval the hall may be freely ventilated and disinfected. The Order applies to every building used as a theatre, music hall, place for public singing, dancing or music place for cinema exhibition or other place of amusement.
>
> To allow half an hour's interval every three hours, one performance a day would be lost, whilst at the houses where the two shows a night principle is in vogue, the first performance would have to commence half an hour earlier than at present. In both instances the proprietors believe they will lose money, and already at the more fashionable city halls an advance in prices has been suggested if the Order is enforced.

Cinema opening was restricted to prevent the spread of flu. *Birmingham Gazette*, 21 November 1918.

Science Museum, London/ Wellcome. CC BY

Many potential customers reacted to the apparent likelihood of catching influenza in the cinema by temporarily withdrawing from this pastime. The *Evesham Journal* noted on 2 November that the audiences at the Grand Cinema were apparently depleted by the influenza, although those who risked attendance were rewarded with what was described as an interesting programme which included Becky Floss in a film about the making of the first American flag. With depleted audiences and the pressure of new regulations, some cinema proprietors decided to temporarily close altogether and in Birmingham, reflecting efforts to prevent the spread of the disease, the Medical Officer of Health's Report noted: 'Locally, various handbills were issued. Cinemas were closed. The local press were most helpful in making known from day to day points which were thought to be of general importance.' In Worcester an irate reader wrote to the *Worcester Daily Times* to request the closure of theatres and cinemas in the city forthwith. Noting that the schools had already been closed in much of the city at the beginning of November 1918, she went on to say:

CHAPTER FOUR

Surely there has been enough death, suffering, and mourning caused by this cruel war without allowing an epidemic like this to rage in the city and country and not take every possible means to stay its course. If the Medical Officer has not the power, I take it the Mayor and the Corporation who are the governing body of the city, should do so at once.

The editors pointed out that there was no such authority but suggested children should not be admitted, as children, with some justification, were seen as carriers of influenza.

However, the cinema was also the medium for distributing public information about how to prevent the spread of the disease. For three consecutive nights in early November a Walsall cinema showed an 18-minute public information film with the title *Dr Wise and a Foolish Patient*. This silent film involved the eminent Doctor Wise giving a lecture with diagrams, notice boards and images of germs seen through a microscope and was designed to shock the audience into taking preventative measures to stop the spread of flu. The 'foolish patient' Mr Brown was shown travelling on public transport, walking along crowded streets, meeting friends and going to work in an office while suffering from the first symptoms of influenza. The film explained how through neglecting his influenza symptoms, foolish Mr Brown has caught pneumonia and spread influenza to hundreds of other unsuspecting people he has encountered. The film's message was not only to encourage those with influenza to stay at home in bed but also to behave like Mr Smith, who followed the advice of Dr Wise, to gargle and douche his nose with a lotion of potassium, pomegranate oil and salt. It was also suggested that anyone interacting with those who had influenza should wear a muslin facemask.

By December as the epidemic began to wane, there was exasperation that some of the regulations and restrictions remained in place for cinemas. Nevertheless, the *Evening Dispatch* in Birmingham argued, on December 19, that despite the reduction in the death rate the influenza epidemic remained serious and there was therefore 'still every necessity and justification for all the precautions taken by the Medical Officer of Health to prevent the disease spreading'. In January there was at last a respite from the virus and the consequent restrictions but not for everyone. Ellen Gibbs of Lower Moor, near Pershore in Worcestershire recorded in her diary: 'Saddened to hear that Mrs

CHAPTER FOUR

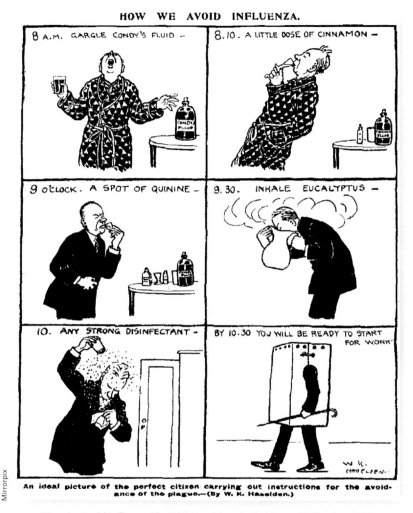

'How to Avoid Influenza' by W K Haselden, *Daily Mirror*, 25 October 1918.

Morris of Hill Furze had died from the Spanish flu. The poor soul had seen all her five sons serve in the Army throughout the war and then, finally, when the anxious years of waiting were over, the influenza claimed her.'

Some parts of the West Midlands escaped the third wave of influenza entirely; while it was not as virulent as that which occurred in autumn 1918, this does not mean that there were no deaths. Coventry had 463 fatalities from influenza in 1918 and only 40 in 1919. Some families like the Ackworths in Malvern heard of loved ones who had died abroad waiting for the long slow process of demobilisation to bring them home. Major D. H. Ackworth had died

CHAPTER FOUR

of pneumonia following influenza in Egypt on 6 February 1919. To many people's dismay, having suffered from influenza in 1918 did not seem to guarantee immunity in 1919.

In the West Midlands in 1919 the experience of the pandemic was shaped by a legacy of fear created by the high death toll that influenza had already exacted the previous year. In Birmingham the third wave of influenza reached its height in March 1919. *The Times* noted on 11 March: 'In Birmingham it is believed to be decreasing in prevalence' and went on to explain that influenza is 'much easier' with 140 deaths the previous week, compared to 157 the week before. Amongst the deaths was 22-year-old Edith Lizzie Haines from Wyre Piddle, Worcestershire who died of influenza whilst working as a servant in the Birmingham suburb of Edgbaston. And Mrs Sutherland, the Colonel of Midlands Battalion of the Women's Volunteer Reserve, also died of influenza and her funeral service took place in Birmingham Cathedral. In Dudley the newspapers reported that the influenza was nearly gone in the borough, but deaths from the virus continued to be recorded in May and June. News also reached the Black Country of the death of William Anderson, who had been MP for Sheffield Attercliffe until 1918. He was the husband of the wife of Mary Macarthur, who had led the Cradley Heath Chain Makers to victory in a strike for a minimum wage in 1910, when she was the general secretary of the Women's Trade Union League, and unsuccessfully stood as a Labour candidate in Stourbridge, Worcestershire in 1918.

Kidderminster also struggled to combat the third wave of this disease; for example, local residents Mr and Mrs Helliwell died within a few hours of each other due to the influenza in March. Reports in the Kidderminster newspapers noted that there were 28 cases of infectious disease, including 22 cases of pneumonia in early April. The Staffordshire Potteries towns were also hit again in March, with 43 dying in one week. Likewise sanitary inspectors reported that schools were closed at Spetchley and Eckington in Worcestershire and that the epidemic was becoming very bad at Pershore, whilst Bewdley also had a good many cases but no deaths in April 1919. Rural Herefordshire also experienced this wave of influenza. The diary entries of Ruth Bourne, who was born in September 1865 at Grafton Manor near Bromsgrove, Worcestershire, chart the long struggle that her husband had with influenza. As was so often the case, it was the better off who were more likely to have recorded their experiences or kept any letters and diaries giving personal accounts of the progress of influenza in individual lives and families, although their experiences were in many ways untypical of the wider population.

Ruth Bailey, née Bourne, was one of nine children whose father, Colonel Bourne, was a prosperous country gentleman and one-time Chairman of Herefordshire County Council. Ruth had kept a diary from the age of eight and on 23 March 1919 noted that 'influenza has been again raging all over the world, many deaths from pneumonia have taken place'. She also recorded that the doctors had not found a cure for it, nor did they know how it came about, something that she would see first-hand a month later when her husband was afflicted with the virus. On 20 April Ruth recorded that she and her husband would be spending Easter alone as he was ill with a bad cough and temperature and indeed on Easter Sunday he seems to have spent all day in bed. He was feeling better a few days later and got up, shaved and sat in the dining room. When the doctor visited on 24 April he was optimistic that Edward was on the mend and gave Ruth an order for a bottle of whisky from the local shop. The tradition of consuming alcohol to combat the symptoms of colds and flu was well established and thought to help prevent the symptoms gravitating into something worse, such as pneumonia or bronchitis.

The medical professions endorsed the idea that alcohol, particularly whisky or brandy, could cure influenza; likewise that the administration of small quantities of brandy at the critical stage in pneumonia often saved lives. However, both beverages were in short supply, restricted by wartime regulations on alcohol consumption. There were demands that stocks that had been prevented from release during the conflict should now be distributed and that government controls over the supply of alcohol should be abandoned. The civil population was, however, not provided with any increase in quantity of alcohol by a government that was led by a Prime Minister who had sympathy with the non-conformist temperance traditions. The Royal College of Physicians was of the opinion that 'Alcohol invited disaster' but many ignored this approach and in London the Savoy Hotel created a new cocktail, which contained whisky and rum and was named the Corpse Reviver. In the West Midlands a good deal of anger was properly displayed at the non-release of what was rightly or wrongly regarded by responsible medical practitioners as a necessity for the saving of life.

In April 1919 Ruth was able to obtain the whisky she required from the

CHAPTER FOUR

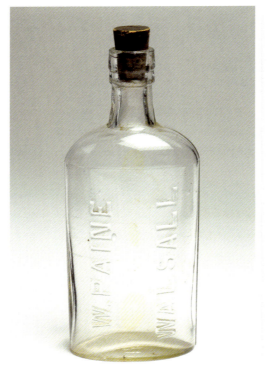

Whisky bottle used by "W. Paine Walsall" to contain 1/- worth of whisky, used for medicinal purposes to combat flu.

local shop, thanks to a certificate provided by the family doctor; without it, she noted, 'whisky was fearfully hard to get'. In November the previous year a friend had turned up, 'quite distressed' wanting whisky as her husband and maid both had the influenza but were unable to obtain it. Others were not so lucky and according to the *Bromsgrove, Droitwich and Redditch Weekly Messenger* in March 1919, Redditch Urban District Council were exasperated by the failure of the government to ensure that sufficient supplies of alcoholic spirits were released 'in order to meet the needs of people who were suffering from influenza'. The council pointed out that in cases of pneumonia it was the opinion of 'the medical profession that brandy and whisky were extremely useful'. Having obtained the necessary whisky, Ruth recorded in her diary the following day that her husband enjoyed his lunch, which included some beef tea, rice pudding and coffee, but he continued to suffer from headaches, a parched throat and had slept all

CHAPTER FOUR

morning. It was nearly two weeks after the original entry that Ruth's final mention of her husband's influenza is recorded on 4 May:

Edward has been quite ill with two distinct attacks of Influenza, and even now he is very pulled down and is glad to stay in bed till lunchtime. Yesterday (May 3rd) he went out into the garden for the first time and felt exhausted and even faint. I was glad to get him home and give him tea after which he revived and Mrs Hall came and played lovely music to him.

As Ruth and her husband were comfortably off, they were able to ensure that the doctor called several times to monitor Edward's progress. This was not the experience of most people in an era when doctors were both busy and expensive and few patients had the benefit of health insurance. Manufacturers' advertising took advantage of people's fears. G. C. Dean, a tailor with premises near the Bull Ring in Birmingham, announced via an advert in the *Handsworth*

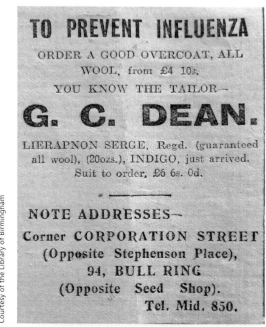

Retailers like G. C. Dean marketed their products on the basis of their ability to combat the flu. Advert seen in the *Handsworth Herald*, 9 November 1918.

CHAPTER FOUR

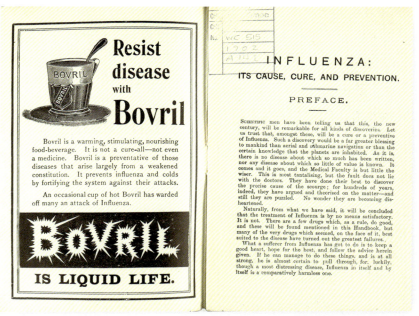

'Bovril is Liquid Life'. Advert and preface to Abel Heywood and Son's *Influenza: Its cause, cure and prevention*, 1902. Bovril was understood to help avoid the flu and aid recovery.

Herald that 'To prevent influenza order a good overcoat all wool from £4 10s' (£4.50). Once again, however, purchasing this extremely costly item was not an option for many families who were surviving on £1–£2 a week. Instead they could purchase 'Myrica tablets made from highly vitalising herbs' or consume a teaspoon of cinnamon oil and quinine every day to prevent themselves catching influenza. Indeed there was concern expressed that the public were 'flying to ammoniated tincture of quinine, and there has been quite a run on this medicine at the chemist's shops by people who have the premonitory indications of a cold'.

Ruth Bourne and her husband could also afford the money to provide the nourishing food and whisky, which were understood to build up his strength. Many others did not have the financial resources to buy such products. There was perhaps no product promoted so strongly to feed those who sought cheap nourishing food as Bovril. The product was visually associated with the strength of a bull, an image of which appeared next to jars of Bovril in its advertising campaigns. During the Russian flu epidemic Bovril was promoted as 'the perfect food for blood, brain and bone' which, when used liberally, would 'fortify' consumers against flu. Indeed Bovril was portrayed in both the Russian and

Spanish flu epidemics as providing the strength to resist influenza and the ability to assist in repairing the body after an attack. For many the struggle to recover from influenza after a severe but not fatal bout of the illness could be lengthy, and Bovril was marketed as assisting this recovery. Lungs or other organs could be permanently impaired, and many doctors in the 1920s and 1930s considered these patients were more susceptible to nephritis, meningitis, encephalitis lethargica and Parkinson's disease.

The importance of Bovril during the 1918-9 influenza pandemic was also linked to the widespread misapprehension that people caught influenza or failed to recover because they were malnourished due to the shortage of meat. Rationing had been introduced in spring 1918, which are allowed individuals only 15oz of meat and 5oz of bacon a week. The low consumption of meat was considered by some to be sapping the vitality of the population. Bovril claimed to have body-building powers and could act as a substitute for meat, which continued to be rationed. So committed was the general population to the almost medicinal virtues of Bovril that shortages occurred. Large adverts in local newspapers encouraged those who could afford to do so, not to stockpile Bovril. Their restraint in purchasing Bovril, it was suggested, would ensure that Bovril could go to the sick. Under the headline *Unselfishness,* one advert explained:

> **There is a simple way of helping others during the present influenza epidemic. It is to refrain from buying Bovril if you have a stock in the house, which will carry you on even for a month. In this way you will leave the available Bovril in the shops for those who have illness at home. Bovril Ltd. recognising that those who are deprived of the body-building power of Bovril may more easily fall victims to the epidemic are doing their utmost to increase the supply.**

Indeed on 7 December 1918 the company took out a large advertisement in the *Evesham Journal* to explain that the shortage of Bovril was due to a shortage of bottles and they were hoping that men would soon be released from the armed forces to work in bottle factories, thereby providing the necessary jars for Bovril. Only two weeks later they felt able to reassure the Bovril-starved residents of Evesham that more Bovril should be on its way to the town in the New Year.

CHAPTER FOUR

Influenza

An Apology for the Shortage of Bovril.

In view of the immense value of Bovril during an Influenza epidemic, the proprietors of Bovril are making every effort to meet the demand. The shortage of bottles is seriously hampering the endeavours to increase the supply, and it is hoped that men will now be released for the bottle factories.

In order that the available supplies may reach those who have most need of Bovril, consumers who already have sufficient Bovril in the house are urged to refrain for the moment from further purchases, except for including in parcels to the front.

The proprietors of Bovril wish to express their regret to all those who have been unable to obtain Bovril in time of need.

Bovril shortages and reassurances that they would soon be over were reported in the *Birmingham Gazette*, 28 November 1918.

Courtesy of the Library of Birmingham

The Registrar General claimed that in the 46 weeks from 23 June 1918 to 10 May 1919 the total deaths attributable to influenza in England and Wales were 151,446, approximately three quarters of which occurred in the second wave. In Birmingham the Medical Officer of Health considered that there were about 400 deaths in the first wave of influenza in June and July 1918, 2,000 deaths in the second wave in November and December, and another 1,400 died between February and March 1919, making a total of 3,800 deaths. Unusually though, he also considered that there were 400 deaths as a consequence of a much milder outbreak in March and April 1920. The flu epidemic in Britain is generally understood to have lasted from 1918 – 1919 and yet the Birmingham Medical Officer of Health and the newspapers were convinced about this 'final bout' in spring 1920.

CHAPTER FOUR

According to the *Birmingham Daily Post* on 16 March 1920, Dr Robertson organised the distribution of 50,000 handbills to the houses of citizens in more crowded areas of the city with advice on preventing the spread of the disease and nursing patients. Prevention included keeping windows open, avoiding crowded spaces and the advice: 'Ask your doctor if he thinks it desirable to vaccinate you against influenza.' An effective vaccination for influenza was not actually developed until 1933 when the flu virus was itself identified. But there were a number of attempts to develop a vaccine before this and a strong rumour emerged that those in the armed forces had been vaccinated whilst those on the home front were left to suffer. Alternatively, there was an unfounded rumour in Birmingham that an inoculation against the virus had been developed in 1919 but was being reserved for doctors and those at public schools.

Less than a week later, in spring 1920, the same newspaper noted that although there was little evidence of an epidemic on the scale of 1918 and 1919, 'there were 33 deaths in Birmingham last week, compared to 150 deaths the same week last year'. The extension of influenza was not thought to be 'alarming at present' but it was considered 'desirable that the citizens should be informed what measures to adopt if influenza does become epidemic'. Coping with the local consequences of this pandemic put a large strain upon the medical service and it is their struggles that the next chapter will address.

CHAPTER FIVE

DOCTORS, NURSES AND THE CHALLENGES OF PROVIDING MEDICAL CARE

A number of doctors and medical students had volunteered at the start of the hostilities and by 1915 a quarter of the profession had joined up. Initially aware of the need to maintain an adequate supply of doctors on the home front, elderly doctors were encouraged back into practice and a number of doctors combined their work with a role in the Territorials. Despite this, at the beginning of 1918, the number of doctors able to minister to patients in the West Midlands was already depleted.

In April 1918, just one month before first cases of influenza were reported in Spain, the British Parliament debated a government proposal to raise the upper age at which doctors could be conscripted into the armed forces to 55. The measure was intended to address the shortage of doctors needed to look after the numerous soldiers with injuries or diseases caused by industrial warfare. The proposal met with much resistance and Sir Auckland Geddes, Minister of National Service, acknowledged that:

> *There are districts in this country where, as the result of the withdrawal of medical men, the supply available is very short, where the young fit man is really necessary, just as necessary as he is in the trenches, and working practically as hard day and night. It is no good talking about putting an old man, who does not know the district and does not know the people, into that position…*

But he reassured the House:

> *We have surveyed the whole country. We have plotted out in every town the number of medical men available and the number of the population whom they may have to look after, and we find that there are in some of the more comfortably off residential cities—not the great manufacturing cities, but cities where you get a retired class—doctors of about fifty, fifty-one, fifty-two, fifty-three and fifty-four who are really in excess of local requirements.*

CHAPTER FIVE

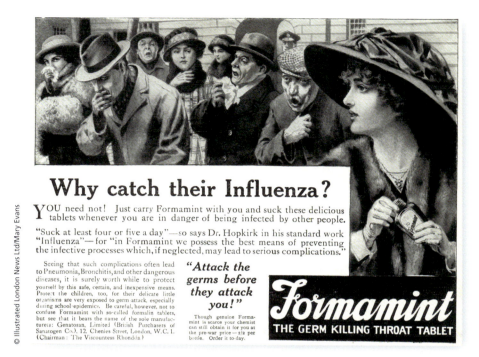

'Why catch their influenza?' An advert for Formamint germ killing throat tablets to guard against the spread of influenza. From *The Sphere*, 16 November 1918, page V and *The Sketch*, 13 November 1918.

The government's proposal was passed and the number of medical professionals on the home front was further depleted – particularly outside the major conurbations such as Birmingham as a result of the priority placed on army medical services. Whilst looking after the health of those actively fighting the war on the battlefront was certainly a national priority, it left the medical facilities at home inadequate to cope with the influenza pandemic. The paucity of doctors severely restricted the care that could be given to those who suffered from the Spanish flu in the West Midlands and quickly led to long queues outside doctors and pharmacies as overworked chemists also tried to plug the need for medical care.

The system of compulsory health insurance, established in 1911, provided sickness benefits in return for a flat rate contribution, the cost of which was shared by employees and employers. Those in regular employment earning less than £160 a year paid 4d (1.5 pence), their employer 3d and the government 2d

CHAPTER FIVE

each week. When sick, contributors received cash payments and limited care from a doctor on a local list or panel and also free treatment for tuberculosis. The doctors were given a standard payment for each panel patient. The unemployed, the elderly, those with irregular employment and dependants, including wives and children, were not, however, covered by this health insurance scheme. If they needed medical care they were compelled to pay for it out of their own pockets. The system should have provided medical care for munitions workers, miners and many of those working in essential war industries in the West Midlands. However, even before the influenza pandemic, the system was already under stress due to both a shortage of doctors and the advanced age of many of those left in practice on the home front. In Droitwich and Hanbury, for example, it seemed impossible to find doctors willing to go onto the panel. Some like Dr Wilkinson felt he was just too old to manage panel work.

Alternatively, Dr Dawes who covered the nearby village of Feckenham and some surrounding areas was preparing to go on active service in the armed forces, and was consequently unwilling to take on patients beyond the areas he was already committed to. Furthermore, he was reticent about travelling up to 5 miles to see a patient in some rural villages. The time taken to travel between patients

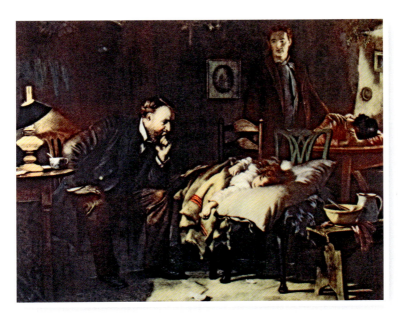

Rural country doctor ponders the fate of a sick child at home as parents look on late at night.

who were often visited in their homes was something of a challenge in 1918. Cars were in short supply, petrol likewise. Many tradesmen's and doctors' horses had been requisitioned for the war effort and whilst bicycles may well have been beneficial for doctors in the relatively flat landscapes of Birmingham and Coventry, they were of limited use in the steep hills in some of the rural areas in Worcestershire, Shropshire and Herefordshire.

Doctors in the West Midlands seem generally to have coped with the first wave of influenza in the summer of 1918. Most patients would not have considered influenza as requiring medical attention at first. A Birmingham doctor with an extensive practice explained to a local newspaper in late June that those cases he had encountered had 'all the usual symptoms of the "flu"...violent headaches, severe pains in the back, extreme prostration and depression' but he had not encountered any 'case of a dangerous type'. The second and more serious wave of influenza between October and December was quite another matter, particularly for those areas that the government had denuded of doctors to supply the army medical services. As the *Worcester Daily Times* reported at the end of October: 'The local doctors, never so short staffed as in recent years, are quite unable to cope with the outbreak though they are working from early morning till midnight. Dr Crowe who is in Birmingham recuperating from an operation, has been away from Worcester for a month, and Dr Bennetts is also unwell. The strain on the remaining medical men is the greater.' Local doctors were apparently working at the highest possible pressure and had never known their services to be in such great demand. Even working 12 or 14 hours a day they were unable to visit all the patients who wanted to see them.

Given the level of medical crisis that the influenza had created, local newspapers were horrified that in late October, doctors were still being called up for military service. The *Worcester Daily Times* noted on 29 October 1918 that doctors were 'busier than they ever have been since the beginning of the war and many are so over-worked that they scarcely have time to eat a meal from breakfast until they finish for the night'. It was not just doctors who were under pressure but also local chemists and one was so hard pressed that he had to ask people to return two hours later to collect prescriptions. Only the wealthiest had telephones to call the doctor and people resorted to desperate measures to try and ensure their loved ones received medical attention. Thanks to newspaper reports and rumour, people were increasingly aware of the speed with which

CHAPTER FIVE

patients could go from relatively mild symptoms of influenza to death. According to the *Worcester Daily Times* on 31 October:

> **Doctor X went on a country round, and soon after his car stopped two or three mothers appealed to him to see their children, saying that they had sent to Dr Y but he had not arrived. In one case a young lady living in a remote district with an invalid mother was removed to a nursing home in order to receive attention.**

The relentlessness of their work during October and November ground down the doctors who by this point were themselves often elderly or deemed unfit for military service. However, light relief came in unexpected forms. Dr Alexander Mackie, who was the works doctor for both Wolseley Motors and the Shell Petroleum Company in Birmingham was approached by a passer-by asking him to look at her pet starling that had broken its leg; he agreed. His relief at being offered, at least momentarily, some respite from treating victims of influenza was so great that this doctor was happy to provide a splint for a lame bird. Whether any doctors were persuaded to look at cats - rumoured to be experiencing their own form of flu that was not infectious to human - remains uncertain.

Dr Mackie may also have been relieved to be able to do something practical and positive for the pet starling: one of the problems that doctors faced in dealing with influenza was the uncertainty of diagnosis and how to effectively treat patients, particularly in the first wave in the summer of 1918. By the early twentieth century doctors had attained a level of professionalism, gravitas and authority, but their credibility must have been taxed by the contradictory opinions held by their own number, as well as by experts and research scientists. Some differentiated between influenza and septic pneumonia - others such as Mr Hayes Fisher, President of the Local Government Board, did not. Nevertheless many doctors appear to have examined patients and been able to report descriptions of their symptoms in minute details - including the speed of the progress of the illness, whether patients were sitting up or coughing, their colour, whether their patients had pains in the head, stomach or elsewhere and whether they ate or not - when giving evidence in coroners' courts. A further problem for some elderly doctors was that they were themselves no longer at

CHAPTER FIVE

their best. After a doctor visited her husband who was suffering from influenza, Ruth Bourne noted in her diary: 'Dear old Dr Prickett came to see him and loved playing at being the doctor again but his memory has got so weak that one can't go by anything he says.'

Doctors prescribed a range of pills, potions and practices, most of which would have been ineffective in attacking a viral disease such as influenza. There

A few more influenza safeguards illustrated, by W.K. Haselden, *Daily Mirror*, 19 July 1918.

CHAPTER FIVE

has even been some speculation that some patients died as a result of over-prescription. Their armory of potential cures included morphine, quinine, strychnine, tobacco, alcohol, hydrotherapy, poultices, blanket baths, camphor injections, soap and water enemas, placing patients in washtubs of scalding water, and cold packs. Some suggested the Malvern Water Cure developed in the mid-nineteenth century in the famous Worcestershire spa town: this involved placing patients on wet beds and sprinkling them with cold water to build up immunity. Alternatively, Ruth Bourne's husband was prescribed 'A new medicine with Sulphate of Soda to get rid of the poison from the influenza'. Despite frequent reports of medical breakthroughs and much talk of bacteria, to the general public 'the overall message, however, was that the medical profession was ignorant of the causes of influenza and powerless to prevent the epidemic'.

The combination of a shortage of doctors and a panic-stricken population from October 1918 onwards created a perfect storm and the strong impression amongst some doctors was that many people were demanding medical attention at the first sneeze. Interestingly, Dr Robertson, the Medical Officer of Health in Birmingham, differentiated between the prevalent and potentially fatal influenza and what he describes as the 'always present condition popularly called influenza cold'. A slight sense of exasperation and even irritation is discernible in the medical profession as October gave way to November and they continued to be run off their feet – sometimes making call to patients with a sniffle and a tickle in their throat whilst others more seriously afflicted insisted on getting up and spreading the influenza far and wide.

There was a growing sense in the guidance being handed out by some to influenza sufferers that perhaps they had contributed to their own demise. The public health warnings were pervaded by a slightly moralistic tone which suggested that influenza was preventable and therefore by implication that it was the patients' own fault if they caught flu. This was reiterated in the medical advice provided in the *Worcester Daily Times* on 25 October 1918:

> **In fact each individual can protect himself or herself by simply "taking care". How many will do so? It is surely the duty of each person to do everything possible to maintain their working capacity in these days of stress when the welfare of the nation depends on everyone doing their best. ….**

CHAPTER FIVE

> Sir Arthur Newsholme in his memorandum wrote as follows: "If every person who is suffering from influenza or catarrh recognized that he is a likely source of infection to others, that some of the persons infected by him may die as the result of this infection, and took all possible precautions, the present disability and mortality from catarrhal epidemics would be materially reduced."

The inadequate medical response to the virus was exacerbated by the episodic nature of the flu and the failure to recognise and deal with its magnitude. Flu was not made a notifiable disease until January 1919, in part because the authorities were aware that there were insufficient doctors to deal with it. Even when the Armistice was imminent and then signed, the government was slow to release doctors from the forces to deal with influenza. Badsey doctor Arthur Sladden wrote to his sister, Kathleen on, 2 November 1918:

> *The war has taught most of us to be cautious and I see and hear very little over-optimism on immediate peace prospects… I'm afraid there's little chance of doctors being released or exchanged for home service. I wish they'd send me over with my lab to do a spell at home. At the moment the great news and prospects keep me going but if the next two weeks prove that the end has receded again I know many of us will inevitably feel a sense of reaction.*

The Armistice came but the shortage of medical personnel did not end and in December 1918 and January 1919 hospitals, municipalities and local communities asked the government to at least temporarily release medical practitioners and nurses from the armed forces, but to no avail. The shortage of medical personnel was exacerbated when they themselves contracted influenza, something that occurred both in general practice and in hospitals.

The vast majority of people in this era prior to the National Health Service would not have chosen to go to hospital to be treated for influenza. Indeed hospital records, for example, for the Infirmary in Worcester, did not necessarily record a high number of deaths from influenza, although there were a number of deaths listed for 'Pneumonia and Influenza'. Nevertheless, hospitals found that they were under pressure in many parts of the region. Birmingham General

CHAPTER FIVE

Hospital and the Infirmaries at Erdington and Selly Oak all banned visiting in July 1918 to try and prevent the spread of influenza inside or outside the hospital. Likewise the *Walsall Observer and South Staffordshire Chronicle* on 13 July 1918 reported: 'The influenza epidemic has been so much in evidence at the Hospital, fourteen cases having developed this week, that it has become necessary for the present to close the wards to visitors.' In November when the influenza crisis was more severe, hospitals were forced to close their doors, both to visitors and to new patients. According to the *Birmingham Gazette,* the General Hospital, the All Saints Asylum in Winson Green and the convalescent homes Glenthorne and Stechford Hall had all closed their doors by the beginning of November.

The three unpredictable waves of the influenza pandemic made it hard to organise special facilities to care for the ill. In some areas, such as Malvern, by the time the authorities had finalised their strategy to provide a temporary hospital, it was spring 1919 and the main threat was over. Some accommodation was made available in the General Hospitals in Birmingham, in the Union Infirmaries and in the City Hospital. Little Bromwich looked after some of the severe cases who could not be cared for at home. Even when special wards in hospitals could be made over to treat the more severe victims of influenza there was a shortage of trained or at least experienced nurses to care for the patients. Too many of them were working with the armed forces, even after the Armistice. It has been suggested that those unable to get to jam-packed hospitals or medical care were most likely to die but efficiency in hospitals was compromised by the tendency of those nurses who looked after influenza patients to themselves catch the virus, even if they were wearing muslin masks over their faces.

The *Worcester Daily Times* reported that local hospitals were suffering severely due to influenza in October 1918 and that 36 nurses and maids had figured on the flu casualty list. Happily none of the cases proved fatal, nor were there any deaths among patients in the hospital from influenza alone. There were, however, fatalities amongst the medical staff of a number hospitals in the region, including Malvern Hospital where several nurses fell victim to the flu. These included Frances Boddington who was 34 when she died on 27 October 1918 and Mr Webb, a 35-year-old blind man, recently married, who worked as a masseur at war hospitals in Birmingham and died after a short bout of influenza. Miss Laura Upton, aged 51 and the Matron of the Corporation Infectious Diseases Hospital in Kidderminster, also died in March 1919.

CHAPTER FIVE

The military hospitals and the hospitals attached to army camps seem to have been particularly badly hit by the virus, perhaps because there were so many people in close proximity to one another, combined with so much to-ing and fro-ing in and out of the hospitals from across the country or abroad. Consequently, nurses working as Voluntary Aid Detachments (VADs) were also victims of the virus as they cared for soldiers when influenza swept through army camps at home and abroad. The Monyhull Colony, a mental hospital for Kings Norton and Aston in Birmingham, had like many similar institutions been used to accommodate a military hospital after the outbreak of the First World War. By 21 November 1918 there were reports of 400 inmates suffering from influenza, 18 members of staff off-duty and 5 deaths.

Miss Lilian Norah Pearce, a VAD at Cannock Chase Military Hospital died, aged 22, on 19 November 1918. Her mother also died 10 days later; both deaths were caused by influenza developing into pneumonia. Canon Owen of

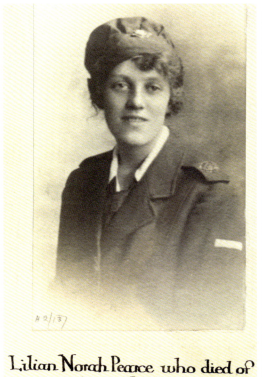

Lilian Norah Pearce died of flu while nursing at Cannock Chase Military Hospital.

Oldswinford near Stourbridge learnt of the death of his youngest daughter Muriel in November 1918. She had been undertaking work as a VAD at Kineton Hospital, Warwickshire where she was one of the youngest VADs in England. On joining Mrs Joshua Fielden's Detachment she had gone to work at Waverley Abbey Military Hospital near Farnham for a short time and then in March 1918 moved to work at the Hôtel des Anglais at Le Touquet, followed by a spell at the Duchess of Westminster's Hospital. When that hospital was closed Muriel returned to work in London at the end of October 1918. She was, however, taken ill and died on 16 November. When her body was returned home for burial, her local church was 'gorgeously decorated with masses of white flowers by members of the congregation' and her coffin was covered with the Union Jack. Cadets Corps sounded the Last Post at the graveside and bells rang a muffled peel at the end of service. Amongst the wreaths were some from the Sisters and Nurses at the VAD hospitals where she had worked. The loss of nurses' lives to influenza whilst caring for the sick in the furtherance of the war effort was sometimes regarded as being on a par with soldiers who lost their lives serving in the military. News reached Uttoxeter, Staffordshire, of a VAD who contracted influenza nursing wounded soldiers in France and died of pneumonia in early November. The Urban District Council announced that 'when the Roll of Honour came to be made of those in the town who had died in the service of their country, Miss Christine Stewart would be included as having sacrificed her life in the same good cause'.

Almost everyone who suffered from the flu, whether it was fatal or not, spent their illness in their homes, hopefully cared for by families or friends. The *Worcester Daily Times* sought to ensure that such patients restrained themselves from drowning their sorrows in an alcoholic stupor. On 31 October 1918 the newspaper carried this suggestion:

> The spread of the disease would be greatly reduced, if persons suffering from it were willing to stay home for a few days. Satisfactory nursing is important in the prevention of complications, and in aiding recovery from a severe attack... Prolonged mental strain, over fatigue, and alcoholism favour the infection; the complication of pneumonia (inflammation of the lungs) is especially fatal among immoderate drinkers.

CHAPTER FIVE

District Nursing Associations, charitable groups that employed district nurses, paying their salaries and providing them with a home, existed in a number of places in the West Midlands region in 1918. Their costs were met from charitable donations, fundraising and sometimes via regular subscriptions paid by members who could then receive nursing care when they needed it. These nursing associations were generally associated with the Queen Victoria Jubilee Institute of Nurses, set up in 1897, which sought to provide training and skills to nurses caring for the poor who were sick. Some District Nursing Associations were linked to the medical care provided by panel doctors under the compulsory medical insurance introduced in 1911. As the influenza virus struck, local authorities were advised to organise 'treatment, nursing and home-help' for influenza-stricken houses and issued a revised circular of advice (with popular leaflets). These impressed upon the public - and on the local authorities themselves - the precautions that preventative medicine suggested were advisable in regard to both protection and treatment.

District Nursing Associations were found to be most valuable in the first wave of influenza when in Birmingham, the Council Health Committee asked the District Nursing Committee to provide more nurses for the poorer class of patients. However, by November when the situation was really severe and the Health Committee again asked the District Nursing Society to provide nurses for the poorer patients and to allocate more of their own nurses to work on care for those with influenza, there were problems. A large proportion of the Queen's Institute trained nurses were performing roles caring for military casualties, either in territorial hospitals or even working in the field. However, there was grave concern in many circles that the absence of skilled nursing in the home may have contributed to high mortality rates. This meant that other medical services and care were curtailed to redirect nursing to looking after influenza victims. For example, infant welfare clinics and visits from health visitors were suspended. There were also a number of largely unsuccessful pleas for volunteers to nurse those with flu in working class areas of Birmingham.

Not everywhere had a District Nursing Association, particularly the more rural areas. So although Warwick, Leamington Spa, Coventry, Brownhills, Chasetown, Southam and Tamworth, for example, were well organised, in other areas the influenza epidemic highlighted the need for nursing care. The Catshill and District Parish Council decided they needed to take action to ensure that a

CHAPTER FIVE

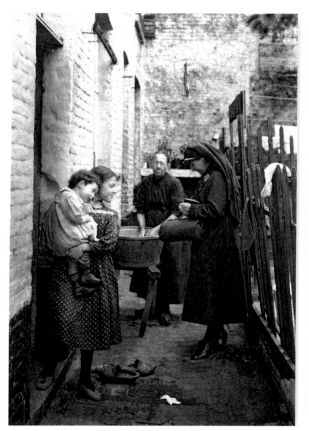

Nurse in dark uniform and carrying a case, visiting a family in her district. A woman is washing clothes in the background and a girl holding a small child stands in a doorway. c. 1910.

nursing association and a district nurse served the area in the future. In November 1918, they formed a committee and an application was made for affiliation to the Worcester County Nursing Association. Assisted by a County Grant of £30, and with pledges of donations from many local people, they were soon on their way towards the £100 needed to obtain the services of a district nurse and trained midwife.

In the absence of adequate district nursing, the responsibility for much of the prevention and nursing of influenza fell on housewives, and the issue was taken up by Margaret Osborne, writing in the *Dudley Chronicle* on 16 November 1918. She pointed out:

CHAPTER FIVE

> It is rather hard luck that an Influenza epidemic should have broken out just now and that we should have a torrent of good advice from doctors on how to avoid Influenza at the very time when there is very little opportunity of taking that advice. To keep warm, to eat good food, and to avoid over-crowding would be easy enough for a good many of us in peace-time, but with rationed food and rationed fuel, and with trains and omnibuses full to bursting we might as well ask for the moon. Moreover, the woman's part – is often to stay at home till someone brings in the influenza and then nurse it. Evidently the very best medical advice is not for us.

By way of support, Bromsgrove medical officers offered housewives nursing the sick assistance in disinfecting clothes. This offer was reiterated in the Worcestershire Medical Officer of Health's monthly report at the end of March 1919, when he pointed out that bedding and clothing could be disinfected at local isolation hospitals for a small charge. However, getting the bedding to the hospital and paying the charge were not inconsequential barriers to many working class women in the district.

The *Evesham Journal* admitted in a report on 2 November 1918 that not only were doctors shockingly overworked but 'nurses were not to be had':

> **At one house in the town the doctor was called in and he found the mother with a baby only a few hours old and in the same room as a little girl and boy suffering influenza. The little girl has since succumbed and the two children have been removed to the Infirmary. Here was this woman in this predicament without help of any sort. We have not heard of any other cases so bad as this, but there are dozens where the mother, although suffering from influenza has had to get about, to the danger of her health to look after her husband and children.**

The dangers to women's health when they undertook the nursing of their immediate or more distant families and friends were constantly attested to in the reports from the coroners' courts in the local newspapers. One woman in the St. John's district of Worcester had apparently succumbed to influenza, after nursing her four children suffering from the same disease, in October 1918.

Edgar Hyde, a rural postman of 7 West Street, Evesham, was the son of a coachman, and also a keen cyclist who had successfully taken part in local competitions prior to joining the wartime army. He was discharged from the forces after being wounded and then in autumn 1918 contracted the influenza virus. His wife, regarded locally as an active and lively young woman in her twenties, nursed him but when she then herself caught influenza she died, leaving him a widower with a child to bring up on his own. The risk of nursing those with influenza was not confined to amateur or inexperienced nurses. Mrs Eliza Sollars from Powick had for ten years been a nurse prior to her marriage and during the war had worked as a VAD, caring for wounded soldiers at Powick Red Cross Hospital in Worcestershire. Nevertheless, a stay in Gloucestershire to nurse her sister led to her own death from influenza and pneumonia. Likewise, Miss Barnett of Kempsey died as a result of contracting influenza whilst devotedly nursing her brother who also died of the disease, leaving their family to cope with a double bereavement in November 1918.

In so many different ways the influenza epidemic brought into the spotlight the inadequacies of medical care in the West Midlands region. The difficulties of trying to provide medical care for the sick during the severe second wave of influenza between October and December and the justified fears of another epidemic led, in Birmingham, to demands for an enquiry to be held at a national level. On 18 December 1918, the Town Clerk wrote to the Local Government Board:

Sir

The Public Health Committee of this city has asked me to represent to the Local Government Board the urgent necessity that exists for an exhaustive enquiry into the whole circumstances of the recent epidemic of Influenza in this country, and into the best means of prevention, which can possibly be adopted.

Approximately 3,000 people have lost their lives in Birmingham during the two epidemics. Of these a large proportion were healthy young adults whose lives were cut off within a few days. No such

CHAPTER FIVE

catastrophe to the public health has occurred since statistical records have been kept and the Committee are advised that from the literature on the subject there is a fear that further reoccurrences of the same disease may be expected.

There is considerable public alarm due largely to the fact that the medical profession itself appears to be in ignorance of the best methods of treatment, and that no assurance can be given as to the steps which are effective in preventing another disaster.

The Public Health Committee feel that such questions as notification, isolation, the use of masks, the use of prophylactic vaccines and of curative vaccines should be taken into consideration by the ablest men whom the country can employ, with a view to defining the best methods of prevention and treatment.

The Public Health Committee therefore respectfully request that the Board will institute the necessary enquiry at the earliest possible date,

I am sir
Your obedient Servant
(signed) J. W. BEAUMONT JONES
Town Clerk

CHAPTER SIX

CONSIDERABLE INCONVENIENCE AND THE BUSINESS OF DYING

As the *Birmingham Mail* noted on 18 November 1918: 'The sudden and large increase in deaths due to the influenza has brought considerable inconvenience in its train and funerals are considerably delayed.' For people working in some occupations – funeral directors, gravediggers and vicars – the pandemic increased their workload to a previously unimaginable level. At the end of 1918 the Registrar General's figures for the 2,118 deaths in Birmingham in relation to occupation suggested that the pandemic had touched many areas of society. The illness and resulting absenteeism and death had created problems in maintaining much of the infrastructure of everyday life across a region already battling with the removal of so many men into the armed forces.

Occupation	Influenza Deaths
Children	492
Housewives	348
No Occupation (females)	362
(males)	16
Labourers	69
Munitions Workers	63
Clerks	63
Brass Workers	50
Iron and Steel Workers	34
Other Metal Workers	42
Shopkeepers	42
Motor Drivers, Carters, etc	36
Domestic Servants	33
Tool Makers	24
Engineers	23
Building Trade	19
Gun Trade	19
Rubber Workers	13
Nurses	11
Publicans, Barmen etc	8
Teachers	7
Professional Men	7
Bakers	6
Blacksmiths	4
Miscellaneous	327

CHAPTER SIX

Industries experienced the disturbance caused by influenza in a variety of ways. For example, the railways were key for the transportation of goods, services and personnel during the war. However, they were also an ideal method for spreading influenza, and this created problems and challenges both for those who travelled on trains and for those who worked on the railways. In October 1918, for example, it was becoming a struggle to keep the railway and station running in Burton-on-Trent, because so many employees were absent through illness. Other areas also lost trained workers. Mabel Rippington was one of 50,000 women employed by the Great Western Railway (GWR) in 1918, cleaning the trains, working in stations as ticket sellers and guards, and donning the distinctively feminine uniform which had an impractically long skirt. Wearing the rather more utilitarian trousers that men wore would have risked displaying women's ankles and was therefore deemed unsuitable. Her husband, Bombardier Rippington, had worked for GWR in Kidderminster prior to the conflict, but by 1918 he was a soldier in France. When Mabel became ill her husband was granted leave to come and see her, but within days of returning to the front he received the news that she was dying. He was, however unable to

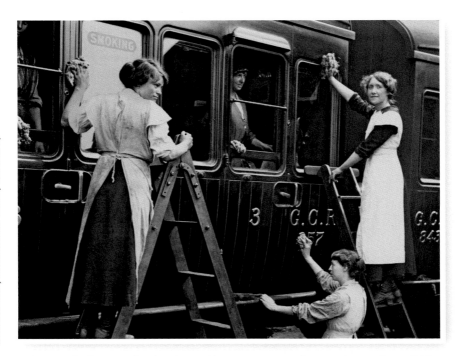

Photograph of women cleaning the smoking compartment of a steam locomotive, c. 1918.

CHAPTER SIX

return and see her again prior to her death or to attend the funeral. When he was finally discharged from the army, he would be denied the chance of fulfilling the dream of so many men at the front – a home and family. His wife of only fourteen months had died and the days they spent together could probably be counted in single figures.

Many men left their jobs on the railways to fight, but as railways were so important in providing transportation for the war effort, a number of workers avoided conscription. Mrs Gardiner of Magpie Lane, Evesham, must have been relieved that her husband, although only in his thirties, had had for many years an important position in the divisional superintendent's office of the GWR and therefore was not required to risk his life in the trenches. However, on the day that the nation was celebrating the Armistice and when many wives were breathing a sigh of relief that their husbands had survived, Mr Gardiner came home from work suffering from influenza. Despite a visit to the doctor and the care that his position and finances could allow, he died one week later leaving her a widow with two young children. There was apparently a very large attendance of railway officials at his funeral, testifying to the 'high esteem in which Mr Gardiner was held'.

He was not the only railway worker to catch the influenza, a number of other railway workers contracted the flu whilst serving in the forces. Lance Corporal Salisbury left his job as a station porter for GWR in Shipton-on-Stour in May 1915 to join the Royal Engineers. After having served in Egypt and France in spring 1919, he left Le Havre bound for Southampton. When he arrived at the demobilisation depot in England on 16 March, he was identified as sick and transferred to hospital. His parents were sent for but he died on 27 March leaving a fiancée, Miss Joyce Sands, yet another couple whose happiness was destroyed not on the battlefields but by a pandemic.

Despite absenteeism and fatalities, the railways did continue to function, along with the police force and the courts of justice, but for these areas of work already stretched by the war, influenza could be very challenging. In West Bromwich the illness of the recorder at the Quarter Sessions forced the closure of the court and the postponement of cases in November 1918. In the same month it was discovered that policemen in some areas were having their wages cut when they were off sick with influenza. This caused some consternation, as reported by the *Evening Dispatch* in Birmingham. Sir Nevil Macready,

CHAPTER SIX

Commissioner of the Metropolitan Police, strongly disapproved of this practice and pointed out the folly of such an action as men needed good food to help them get over the flu. The police force interacted with a wide range of the general public and it is not surprising perhaps that the newspapers were peppered with reports of deaths from among their ranks. These included, in November 1918, 49-year-old George Smith, the Chief Constable of Kidderminster, who had previously worked for Oxford City Police Force. Detective Sergeant Handley died in Worcester after a 10-day illness. He left a wife and four children, one of whom was in the Royal Flying Corps. He had come to Worcester from West Bromwich in 1903 and earned a merit badge for arresting a man for robbery with violence on Pitchcroft in the city in 1913.

Members of the clergy from all denominations also discovered that the pandemic significantly added to their workload. To a greater or lesser degree the majority of the region's population were Christian in one form or another and especially at moments of crisis. Like the medical profession, clergy numbers were also depleted by the war; although they were not conscripted for combative service many clergy of all denominations did feel that it was their duty to serve alongside or minister to their men on the battlefront. The Reverend E. M. Poole held a pastorate for the congregational church in Malvern in 1911 but in the first years of the war he tried unsuccessfully to enlist several times, only to be rejected on medical grounds. In 1917 he spent four months working in an unoccupied corner of Belgium for the Young Men's Christian Association. He returned to work for the YMCA again in 1918, this time in France. When he left Malvern, the other teachers and scholars at the Holly Mount Sunday School presented him with a fountain pen, little realising they would never see him again. He died in France of pneumonia following influenza on 31 October, leaving a widow, a child and a widowed mother.

Clergy on the home front were also expected to visit the sick, and the majority of the population - even if they were not regularly attending church - would have expected religious leaders to perform funerals and remembrance services and to visit the bereaved. Most Irish Catholics living in Birmingham would also have wanted a priest to administer the last rites to their sick loved ones. In January 1919 a *Bishop's Letter* published in the Church of England parish magazine for Bradely and Church Eaton, Staffordshire, noted that the clergy:

CHAPTER SIX

During these past weeks have had the most serious work in visiting the victims of the influenza epidemic and ministering to their bodily and spiritual needs. In many places they have had little rest by day or night. No true parish priest ever fears infection, but the labour and anxiety have been trying to the extreme.

For some religious leaders the sacrifice was not merely of their time and labour, but also, as the local newspapers reported, of their lives to influenza, no doubt contracted from their parishioners, whilst for others overwork led them to neglect other duties. One overworked vicar in Coventry left two couples who were expecting to be married waiting at the altar on an April afternoon in 1919. Between visiting those sick with influenza, the numerous requests for weddings that followed the return of many men from combat, and his vicarage having been let to a munitions factory and not yet returned, the vicar was evidently all at sixes and sevens and had forgotten the young couples' nuptials.

For those who were, so to speak, in the business of death the sudden increase in fatalities brought both potential financial rewards and an unparalleled and often unmanageable demand for their services. The crisis was at its most acute by November 1918 when a reporter in Coventry noted that 'one cannot walk along the main roads leading to the cemeteries without witnessing a funeral procession'. In Kidderminster, there were 40 funerals in five days and in Chipping Campden, three or four funerals every week. Funeral

> **FIVE IN ONE HOUSE DIE.**
> At Burton-on-Trent three members of a family—father, mother, and child—were removed to the workhouse infirmary, and all died within a couple of days, while there were already two children lying dead in the house before they were removed.
> In another case, no one had been seen about an isolated house for three days, and as a dog was heard whining an entrance was effected. It was found that the entire household of three persons were so ill that they were unable even to summon help, and one of them subsequently died.

Death of a family in Burton-on-Trent reported in the *Birmingham Gazette*, 3 December 1918.

CHAPTER SIX

directors were described as 'at their wits' end' to know how to cope with the massive increase in demand for their services. One local firm apparently carried out an average of eighty funerals a week during the last three weeks of November 1918 in Birmingham.

Burying the victims of influenza with the appropriate degree of ritual to convey respect to the dead, as expected in that era, became increasingly difficult. The Victorian and Edwardian funeral is often understood to have been an elaborate and extravagant affair: it was hugely varied according to the wealth, social status and class of the family of the deceased. There was a multitude of different ways in which those who had died were mourned and their bodies disposed of. At one end of the spectrum was Queen Victoria's elaborate funeral in 1901, which she had planned herself and involved more troops than the British Expeditionary Force that initially went to France in 1914. For the poverty-stricken there was a pauper's funeral, paid for by the local authority and involving unceremonious burial in an unmarked and sometimes mass grave.

In Edwardian Britain, funerals served to turn private grief into a public ritual, to mark the significance of the deceased's life and their family's respectability. Funeral collections, the funeral procession and the wake or funeral tea all enabled communities to participate in the mourning and support the bereaved. The arrangements for the funeral, drawing curtains or black shutters on the house of the deceased, the wearing of black clothing by the families, all signified respectability. It has been suggested that the sheer scale of death in the First World War and the decision not to repatriate the dead, leaving their families with no body to bury, was responsible for a cultural change to the rituals associated with death and mourning in Britain. This downplays both the significance of the influenza pandemic and the changes that were already taking place to the practices and rituals of death in Victorian and Edwardian Britain. However, the idealised Victorian death scene familiar from melodrama and popular fiction, where the dying lay peacefully in their own home able to say goodbye to family and friends, became impossible both for those who died on the battlefields and for many who died during the influenza pandemic.

Some of the ways in which wartime shifted practices of death were a consequence of the shortage of manpower in funeral and burial businesses as men joined the armed forces. Although undertakers were acknowledged as an important profession; while some were able to avoid conscription, others were not.

CHAPTER SIX

The number of men employed as undertakers in Birmingham was reduced from 190 in 1914 to only 90 by 1918. Gravediggers, who by definition had to be fit and fairly young men, were likewise conscripted into the army in significant numbers. In April 1918 Mr James Tart, for the Estates Committee of the Corporation, explained to a military tribunal in Birmingham: 'It was in the interests of the health of the city that the staffs of the various city undertakers should not be further depleted. If the undertakers could not bring the bodies to the cemeteries they could not be buried, and there would be a danger of an epidemic.' He went on to argue that 'the matter was one of utmost importance to the health of the city'. Before the year was out the dangers he had warned about came true: there was an epidemic and bodies were unable to be buried.

Prior to the war, radical reformers were already criticising the expense of many of the practices of mourning. There was some condemnation of what was perceived to be working class extravagance and unnecessary expenditure on funerals. Some reformers joined the Cremation Society of England, which had been formed in 1884 to promote both the social acceptance and wider practice of cremation. These included Frederick Lehmann who was briefly elected MP for Evesham, Worcestershire in 1880. Birmingham was the ninth city to build a crematorium when it opened its facility at Perry Bar in 1903. However, much prejudice against the practice remained and with fewer than 1,300 people cremated across the whole of Britain in 1914, this option was only going to be of limited assistance in resolving the problems that were created by the influenza pandemic in the region.

Undertakers were already curtailing the services they offered by the summer of 1918, due to the shortage of manpower and the materials needed for funeral paraphernalia. There was a shortage of timber for coffins, horses for the cortège, and black fabric to make mourning dress or curtains for houses. By the same token, the rise in the death rate from influenza led many undertakers to put two rather than four horses on a funeral carriage and to stop the practice of polishing the wood on coffins. There were appeals for people to tone down their demands for pomp and performance in rituals of death, and for volunteers with horses and vehicles to lend them to the funeral directors. The *Birmingham Daily Post* reported on 15 June 1918 that, at a meeting of the Birmingham Horse and Vehicle Owners Association, undertakers had unanimously decided

CHAPTER SIX

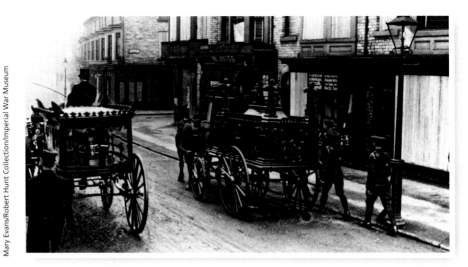

Funeral of Driver Bennett RFA who was killed during a German air-raid on Scarborough, England, during First World War, December 1914.

not to send out more than two horses with each hearse and also not to fix black shutters to windows after deaths were announced.

The prohibitive cost of funerals was a major issue for many working class families: funeral directors were seen as profiteers by some and a large number of local newspaper adverts from funeral directors promoted their services on the basis of the reasonably-priced, fixed-cost funerals that they offered. For example, Brookfield (Successors) Ltd, undertakers in Lichfield Road, Birmingham explained to potential customers that they could carry out funerals efficiently and inexpensively. The desire to avoid the ignominy of a pauper's funeral led many to take out funeral insurance, and these companies, like life insurance companies, found the second wave of influenza financially very challenging. The Prudential, whose representatives called on many West Midlands homes to collect weekly insurance premiums, claimed they were called on to pay out more money during October and November 1918 than even during the period of most intensive fighting and wartime casualties. Charities and neighbours trying to provide the customary financial support to families or help with funerals costs could not cope with the increased demands placed upon them by so many sudden deaths. For example, Maxwell Bullivant's grandparents both died from influenza and, like so many people, were buried in paupers' graves at Brandwood End cemetery in Birmingham.

CHAPTER SIX

However, according to a prominent Birmingham undertaker, writing in the *Birmingham Daily Post* on 15 June 1918, there was no evidence that as a result of either the war or influenza, the public wanted to save expense on funerals. He claimed that 'the outlay had been limited only by the conditions that the undertakers themselves been obliged, owing to the scarcity of labour, to impose'. With the customary criticism of working class expenditure on funerals, which did after all keep him in business, he went on to add: 'At many of the funerals amongst the better class the coffins were of unpolished oak, and for his part he thought all coffins might be unpolished and a great deal of labour saved, thereby; but many of the working class would have the coffin polished.' Despite this undertaker's opinion, working class families and communities did often search for ways of showing respect without the expense of the full regalia of mourning clothes and a costly funeral. Men would wear a black tie rather than a black suit, women wore black or dark items of clothing for a shorter time than once they had, and in rural districts wild and garden flowers were placed on the coffin or grave as a mark of respect rather than shop-bought wreaths.

Where a family suffered more than one fatality in a short space of time, the deceased often shared a funeral and sometimes even a coffin. When Robert and John Allwood of Market Drayton, Shropshire, died from influenza on the same day in November 1918, they had a joint funeral. The report of the event indicates another reason to curtail mourning or the holding of an elaborate funeral tea or wake. As influenza often hit whole families, a number of people in the family were often unable to attend their friend's, sibling's or partner's funeral as they were themselves suffering. Furthermore, a home with members of the family lying sick in bed with influenza did not make a hospitable place to hold a funeral tea. Robert and John Allwood's mother and two of their sisters were laid up with influenza and unable to take on their role as mourners. The problems of arranging funerals also made widespread attendance difficult to manage. In the past, working class families had often chosen to hold funerals on Sundays so that people could attend without the expense of taking a day off work. During the huge demand for funerals in the worst months of the pandemic, families often had to accept any funeral slot they were offered, whether or not others could attend.

It was the inner cities which seemed to struggle most to manage the volume of funerals required. In rural areas agricultural workers could perhaps be utilised to dig graves. Nevertheless, the stress on undertakers did seem to have an impact in many parts of the region. According to the *Worcester Daily Times* on the 11 November 1918, a hearse overturned after colliding with a tram in London Road, Worcester, leaving the overworked and strained driver in a state of shock and needing the services of the doctor. The peak in volume of fatalities in Birmingham in November 1918 created the severest problems and neither funeral directors nor gravediggers could cope with the demand for their services. Young lads below conscription age or those who were too old to fight could not easily remedy the shortage of fit young men to dig graves. Interestingly, there does not seem to have been a suggestion anywhere that women should take on the job of gravedigging, despite them having taken on many other previously male roles. As the death toll rose in 1918, West Bromwich funeral directors were delaying funerals owing to the insufficient availability of mourning coaches in early November. As dead bodies waited for burial in homes and mortuaries, funeral directors began to bolster their promotional rhetoric by advertising not only the cheapness of their services but also their ability to come and fetch bodies at speed, by day or night and even on Sundays. Some even offered guarantees about how quickly they would attend to corpses.

By mid-November, the *Birmingham Daily Gazette* noted the Lord Mayor's concern that delays in funerals were leading to dead victims of influenza remaining in houses and sharing rooms with the living. In Edwardian Britain it was traditional for the dead to remain at home for one or two days, sometimes with the coffin open for friends and family to come and pay their respects. However, the influenza cut across such traditions, and where there were other members of the household suffering with influenza, visiting the house may well have been regarded with some trepidation. Furthermore, the particularities of the Spanish flu and the heliotrope cyanosis that patients suffered could lead their bodies to discolour in a fairly gruesome way, sometimes even appearing black. The situation had become so severe in Birmingham that news of it reached the national newspapers. *The Times* noted on 27 November 1918:

> **The heavy death toll in Birmingham… is placing a great strain on the undertakers and gravediggers. The Lord Mayor stated yesterday that he was 'informed that in many cases dead bodies remained in**

small houses, and in some instances are in the rooms occupied by the living.' He had 'taken steps to secure the additional labour required' from the military and to 'have the bodies removed to some suitable repository until they can be interred'. 594 deaths in Birmingham last week, compared to 475 the previous week.

INFLUENZA EPIDEMIC IN BIRMINGHAM.

DIFFICULTIES IN THE BURIAL OF THE DEAD.

The increasing number of deaths due to influenza and respiratory diseases is placing a heavy strain on the undertakers in Birmingham. Their staffs have been so depleted by the war that it was often very difficult for them to fulfil their instructions in normal conditions, but now the demand upon their services is so great that frequently many days elapse before it is possible for interments to take place. This naturally occasions much distress to the relatives of the deceased persons, and the matter is so serious that action is now being taken by the authorities to ensure more prompt burial. Upon this point the Lord Mayor (Alderman Sir David Brooks) said in the course of an interview yesterday:—"I am informed that in many cases dead bodies remain in small houses, and in some instances are in the rooms occupied by the living. This is a state of things which cannot be allowed to continue, and I have taken steps to secure the additional labour required through the military and from other sources, and also to have the bodies removed to some suitable repository until they can be interred. It is only fair to say that the undertakers and the Estates Committee of the City Council, which is the Burial Authority, are fully alive to the urgent importance of this matter, and are taking all measures possible to remove the existing difficulties."

Newspapers noted the difficulties of burying victims of flu, as here in the *Birmingham Post,* 27 November 1918.

CHAPTER SIX

Civic action was finally taken to deal with the crisis. In Birmingham, military troops were brought in to assist in removing bodies and digging graves; in Coventry soldiers likewise helped to dig graves and in Wolverhampton the local authority ordered the cemetery to extend its opening hours and be open as early and as late as practically possible. The *Birmingham Daily Post* was soon able to announce that:

> **Disposal of the dead has shown 'marked improvement, thanks to the arrangements made by the authorities'. Only two days' notice is required for a public grave in a cemetery. The only issue is the provision of horses and drivers. The military has been asked to provide horses and men.**

A volunteer corps of citizen drivers were recruited and allocated to the various undertakers by the local authority to ensure that the volume of funerals could be catered for.

National as well as local government needed to take action; the problems of dealing with corpses of influenza victims exasperated the population who were already irritated about what they saw as the slow release of men from the armed forces after the Armistice. There were demands made in Parliament that those men who had the necessary skills to help construct coffins, manage funerals and dig graves should be released as soon as possible, given that an armistice had been declared.

Influenza was in other ways intimately linked with the repatriation of soldiers and the transition to peace. Indeed, the management of the death and funerals of soldiers laid bare some of the difficulties and tensions that existed around the care of those who served in the armed forces. The families of men discharged from the forces who died of their injuries at a later date were able to receive a grant of up to £5 to cover their funeral costs. The *Birmingham Daily Post* noted on 21 December 1918 that the administrators for the Birmingham Citizens Committee (which looked after and supported veterans) had received 178 applications for funeral grants in 1918. It assisted in 104 cases at cost of £296 10s (£296.50), approximately £3 per funeral. This high figure, which they struggled to pay out, was understood to be a consequence of high death rates amongst the wounded who had contracted influenza on their return home.

CHAPTER SIX

The families of those who received such grants were in some respects the lucky ones.

The Birmingham Citizens Committee did not respond favourably to grant applications towards funeral expenses for the dependants or widows of discharged men who died of influenza. Nor when they had considered the matter were the Committee of the opinion that they would 'be justified in urging the Ministry of Pensions to extend their regulations to allow them to cover such cases or give assistance out of local funds'. What could be seen as a hard-hearted approach to these victims of the flu was no doubt shaped by the awareness that the Ministry of Pensions and all charitable servicemen's welfare bodies were already reeling under the high costs of supporting so many widows and families of the war-dead and paying their pensions. However, it must have seemed very hard that, as a consequence, those who had fought for their country for four years, or the widows who had lost their husbands in the First World War, were often obliged to have a pauper's funeral. It sent out a very bitter message in a culture in which funerals were very much seen as a marker of the value of someone's life. It was another example of how the consequences of the pandemic were inextricably tied up, for many of the population, with the trials of war.

CHAPTER SEVEN

Schools and the young

Unlike the seasonal influenza that occurred every winter, the fatalities from the Spanish flu were most likely to be young adults, not the elderly or the young. This does not mean the impact of the pandemic on children's lives was minimal, quite the reverse. For example, 492 children died of influenza in Birmingham in 1918, many others became orphans as a result of the pandemic and numerous children had their homes, schooling and pastimes disturbed in a multitude of different ways by the influenza. These included the singing of the following nursery rhyme by schoolchildren:

> *I had a little bird*
> *Its name was Enza*
> *I opened the window*
> *And in-flu-enza*

One of the quirkiest of the interferences the virus brought to children's culture was 'the famine in juvenile picture papers' reported in the *Worcester Daily Times* on 4 November 1918. This was a consequence of so many children in the city being ill with influenza that there was a 'rush for the periodicals, which are a joy to the little ones'. Parents and friends created an unprecedented demand for the magazines which were used to amuse children who were confined to their bed by the illness. The challenges, changes and disturbance to children's lives caused by influenza came at a time when their schooling had already been disrupted by war and in the West Midlands region, like the rest of the nation, there was much concern over child welfare.

The death of so many young men on the battlefields and the poor fitness of many potential army recruits encouraged social reformers right across the political spectrum to see not only the preservation of infant life but also an improvement in children's health as issues of national concern during wartime. High infant mortality figures caused apprehension; the Bishop of London pointed out that while nine soldiers died every hour in 1915, to too did twelve

CHAPTER SEVEN

babies. Thus it was more dangerous to be a baby living in the slums than a soldier on the Western Front. The issue of infant mortality was seen by some as a commercial opportunity and the *Birmingham Daily Mail* carried adverts for Scott's Emulsion which, like the Bishop of London, reminded mothers that during the first fifteen months of war more children were carried away by weakness and disease than British soldiers were killed in conflict. Throughout the war activities to improve infant welfare mushroomed and included a multitude of ways of encouraging and educating working class mothers, including holding annual baby weeks. Local newspapers carried images and reports of baby shows, such as one organised in Kidderminster, where the almost 400 entrants were all given 'bibs' whilst the winners in various age categories received war savings certificates. Across the region local authorities, charities and do-gooders sought to run maternal and child welfare clinics, often in cooperation with District Nursing Associations. The notoriety of the

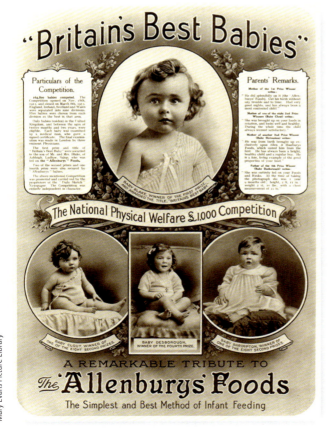

Best Baby Competition. Advert in the *Illustrated London News*, 14 March 1914.

do-gooding women who visited working class mothers in Stoke-on-Trent reached the pages of Scottish newspapers where it was claimed that trained midwives had requested the visits of these 'zealous often autocratic meddlesome ladies, might be postponed until the tenth day', adding: 'The habit of these ladies is to descend on the hapless mother when her baby is a day old, armed to the teeth with lectures, pamphlets and even scales.'

Influenza put a halt to these activities intended to improve infant welfare: for example, maternal and infant welfare clinics were cancelled at Bromsgrove, Oathill and Rubery to prevent the spread of disease. District nurses and volunteers were reallocated to care for those suffering with influenza. A much greater problem for those seeking to replace 'the lost generation' of the young killed on the battlefields was the tendency for pregnant mothers who caught influenza to miscarry or go into premature labour. It is impossible to estimate how many young lives never came into being because of influenza, as these figures are not recorded. However, in April 1919 the *Evesham Journal* noted that Brailes Rural District Council in Warwickshire had reported an increase in infant and premature deaths as a result of influenza, which statistically represented an infant mortality rate of 461 per 1000. It is also impossible to estimate the degree to which the problems experienced by mothers who had influenza and who were struggling to care for their young babies contributed to rises in infant mortality. There are only glimpses of such tragedies. For example, the *Malvern Gazette* reported that Mrs A. Powell died from pneumonia following influenza, aged only 31, in March 1919. Her son who was only two days old died an hour after his mother and they were both buried in the same grave. There is also no indication of how many children grew up with poor health due to damage caused by a bout of influenza suffered as a child.

The newspapers do provide multiple heartbreaking stories of parents whose children died of influenza. One such case was Margaret Alice McGee, the 5-month-old daughter of William, an engineer's fitter, and his wife Mary Rosina of Shrubbery Road, Worcester.

At the end of October 1918, the *Worcester Daily Times* reported that of the 15 who had died in the city from influenza during the previous week, 9 were children under 14 years old, including a baby of one month and children aged three and four. The details of little ones who died suddenly were provided in newspapers, arguably to encourage other parents to be extra-vigilant in caring for their children. For example, in early October 1918 there was a report of an infant who had been apparently fretful all day, continued to cry at night and also the next day, although his mother was able to feed him. When she went upstairs to see the baby at 9 the next morning he seemed quiet but at 10:30 looked ill. She rushed down to fetch her husband who, on going upstairs, found the infant 'very hot and dead' and called the doctor. There were apparently two other children with influenza in the house but the baby had not been taken to see them. The coroner pronounced that the baby had died of bronchial pneumonia, brought on by influenza.

The assumption, with some justification, that children were likely to catch and spread influenza led to the curtailment of a range of their activities. In many parts of the region, children's homes stopped visits in July 1918. These homes faced an even bigger challenge during the second wave of influenza between October and December later that year. The *Worcester Daily Times* reported on 31 October that all the children in the cottage homes in Worcester were down with influenza. Mrs Farrington, the matron of one of these homes, was in bed for a fortnight with influenza but apparently recovered. In the same week the *Birmingham Daily News* reported that: 'The epidemic has spread rapidly in the Rowley Regis district during the last few days, the victims being chiefly children, amongst whom there have been some deaths. Hundreds of school children are absent and the education authority has decided to close three of the schools for a fortnight.'

Children's education had already been severely compromised by four years of warfare. Their teachers had been recruited into the armed forces to be replaced by elderly teachers brought out of retirement. Lessons were constantly interrupted by activities to support the war effort, such as fund raising, knitting comforts for soldiers or growing vegetables on the playing fields. If they lived in rural areas children also took time out of lessons to gather blackberries to be made into jam for the armed forces. Children of ten and eleven were frequently released from school before the legal leaving age of twelve, so that they could work in the factories and the fields. The local newspapers and the logbooks from schools throughout the region chart the massive, added interruption that influenza brought to youngsters' education.

Schools closed and lessons were restricted, either to stop the spread of infection or because so many teachers were themselves ill, during all three waves

CHAPTER SEVEN

> **MORE SCHOOLS CLOSED.**
>
> The influenza mortality at West Bromwich reached its highest point last week, 61 deaths being registered up to Saturday night. The health authorities are doing all they can in the way of prevention, and also in the provision of skilled nursing.
>
> All the elementary schools are remaining closed for another week, and it has been found necessary to close the secondary schools this week owing to the number of pupils and teachers suffering from the malady.

Numerous schools were closed to prevent the spread of the virus, as reported in the *Birmingham Post*, 3 December 1918.

of influenza. As early as 29 June, the *Birmingham Daily Mail* reported that. J. A. Palmers, Secretary of the City's Education Committee, had declared that Birmingham schools where the disease was rampant would be closed and within two days 200 schools shut their doors. In Smethwick, schools were so seriously affected by the influenza epidemic that the whole education department closed for two weeks in July. Estimates suggested that half the schools in the Birmingham area were shut in July, and where schools were open, parents were instructed not to send their children to school if there was any sign of illness. Some parents chose to keep their children away from school to prevent them catching influenza; others wanted their children in the classroom so that schools could keep them out of harm's way while the parents were at work.

All educational establishments were at risk from influenza. At Birmingham University when students assembled for the autumn term in 1918, they spread the virus among the student body and many fell victim to influenza. A student, simply named 'Flora', wrote a lengthy poem called *A Tragedy – With A Happy Ending* about getting back into the routine of studying after the summer holidays at home. She recounted how:

> *The germs flew around me,*
> *Unwilling to wound me*
> *On minding with the pity the vac, I'd been through*
> *But one I declare,*

CHAPTER SEVEN

Lost its way in my hair
And I discovered I'd harboured the 'flu'.
The exams – coming on,
I – resigned my fate
I prayed to the gods, Olympus was obdurate.
My knowledge packed head
Was as heavy as lead :
How could one expect to get through in that state !

She goes onto explain how avoiding self-pity, she ploughed on undertaking her six hours of exams in a fever which led her to write 'terrible prose'. Despite her anxieties and less-than-perfect performance, she passed and ended her poem announcing:

Now a paean of praise
To the Prof. I will raise
Who so graciously pardoned my faults when I strayed:
Thus in spite of the flu
I am happily through :
You see how the gods love a virtuous maid.

The poem appeared in the Birmingham University students' newspaper *The Mermaid* in November 1918, and the editor's notes comment on the challenges of trying to produce the magazine with so many students suffering from influenza, which had delayed the publication date. In further notes she wants to know: 'Is the outbreak of the "Flu" resultant on the germ and dust

Editorial

At the time of going to press we are sad to see that so many people are falling victims to influenza. This accounts for the shortness of the paper, as many who, no doubt would have sent copy have been otherwise engaged.

Courtesy of Cadbury Research Library, Special Collections, University of Birmingham

From *The Mermaid* - a new magazine produced by the students for the students in November 1918.

infected corners of the rooms' at the University? However, perhaps realising that this might not be a diplomatic line for her editorial, she then crosses it out.

Many schoolchildren's education suffered rather more than Flora's university studies seem to have; when the second wave of influenza became established across the region in autumn, schools began to close again. The *Evening Dispatch* noted on 24 October that 'owing to the influenza epidemic, the Medical Officer of Health has closed all the elementary schools at Redditch'. It was stated that there were a great many cases and several deaths had been reported. Doctor Fosbroke, the County Medical Officer for schools in Worcestershire, was severely taxed rushing around the county inspecting children and closing schools. He extended the closure of Redditch schools until 12 November and also closed schools in nearby Astwood Bank where the head of the Roman Catholic Girls School noted in the logbook 'flu epidemic raging in the village'.

Decisions about whether children should be in school and whether schools should be closed were controversial. Mr F.T. Spackman, Secretary for Elementary Education, wrote to the *Worcester Daily Times* in early November and explained:

> **There is growing up a different opinion amongst medical men as to whether or not it is the best thing to keep the schools open in spite of the epidemic, as children are better in well ventilated schools than in stuffy homes or running about the streets. There is not the same degree of cleanliness when children are playing about at home or in the streets as when they are in schools, and dirt is one of the great means of conveying infection. Therefore if the conditions are sufficiently favourable, on Monday the schools will not be 'closed'.**

Mr F.T. Spackman objected to alarmist statements that if schools were opened again, parents would take the law into their own hands and refuse to allow their children to attend. His reasoning and his statements assumed, in line with the thinking of the time, that influenza was caused by bacteria present in dirty environments, rather than a virus which could be transmitted regardless of the level of cleanliness.

Whatever his views, many schools throughout the region were closed for several weeks in November and December. Furthermore, even when they were open, it was difficult for parents to avoid being alarmist when their children attended the funerals of school friends killed by influenza. When 13-year-old Doris Muriel Ashfield's funeral took place at St Mary's Church at the end of October 1918, teachers and class mates from the Girls' Secondary School in Worcester were present although her elder sister remained at home in Britannia Square, ill with influenza. Despite the views of Mr F.T. Spackman, on 9 November *Berrow's Journal* reported that all Worcester's elementary and Sunday schools were to remain closed for at least another week and that on the 'advice of the Medical Officer, visits to Worcester Workhouse have been suspended, and all children of inmates are being kept from school'. Likewise, schools in Wolverhampton and Dudley were closed in November and in Wolverhampton the lending library and children's department were also shut until further notice on 6 November.

Although private schools were not troubled by the Medical Officer of Health's inspections and instructions, the *Birmingham Daily News* noted on 1 November 1918 that a number of private schools within the city were shut. Boarding schools across the region suffered from the spread of influenza amongst students from across the country, who then lived in close proximity to one another in school dormitories. Cheltenham Boys' School, rather than closing or excluding pupils, locked their students in and forbade them from visiting the local town. Malvern College, Worcestershire, in an editorial in the *Malvernian Magazine* in November 1918, noted that the 'influenza germ produced greater changes here in a week than the Kaiser and his forces in four whole years'. The following year, Mr W. J. Stephenson Peach, in charge of the engineering department at the College, died of pneumonia following a bout of influenza.

Many schools were shut when the Armistice was declared; but for those schools which did manage to remain open in October and November the absence of teachers caused problems, as Hilda Moss recalled:

> *It wasn't as bad in Birmingham as some places but the other children were away from school, my teacher had gone away to nurse her family and I remember we were all, instead of in two or three classrooms, we were all in one classroom. The younger children came along and the*

CHAPTER SEVEN

headmistress left us cos our teacher was away and gave us work and we all sat together in this room and I was a bit old I suppose most of them were a bit younger but I was a you know in charge, to see to it that they were quiet. So, and I remember working away at a French exercise and suddenly the signal went off, they called them the maroons. Some of the explosions at the local police station and that was to be the sign of the Armistice was signed.

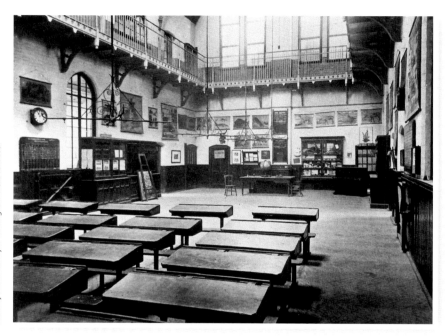

Icknield Street Board School. Hundreds of children had their schooling interrupted by flu.

Indeed the incapacity and death of the teachers made keeping the schools open challenging, even in rural areas. The head of the Girls' Department, Astwood Bank Roman Catholic School, Redditch noted in her logbook: 'Re-opened this morning after being closed for three weeks by order of the County Medical Officer – Dr Fosbroke. School Number now present on books 77. Mistress absent suffering from influenza.' The head of Coventry Street School, Kidderminster recorded: 'the work of the school is somewhat disorganised owing to illness of teachers and scholars.' Young female teachers were a particularly vulnerable group it seems, being in contact with so many viruses at

CHAPTER SEVEN

school and of the age at which fatalities were most likely to occur. Mr and Mrs Jellyman, publicans in Brownhills, would have been distraught to discover their 21-year-old daughter, a teacher at France Lynch School in rural Gloucestershire, had died from influenza. Likewise, Christina Paton, Headmistress of Rye Croft Girls' School in Newcastle-under-Lyme, died in November 1918. In Rugby the Master and Matron of the Workhouse, Mr and Mrs Dickens, also passed away, victims of the virus, in early November.

The virulence of influenza differed from one town to another and even within suburbs and parts of major cities. On 19 November 1918 the *Birmingham Gazette* reported: 'The disease is rife among school children. Several schools were closed last week and yesterday it was decided to close departments in 34 other schools.' Only the day before a more nuanced report in the *Birmingham Mail* claimed that elementary schools and education departments were closed and that the disease was most prevalent on the south side of the city. However, it also argued that school attendances had not been so seriously affected as during the summer epidemic. At this point, in the latter half of November, schools in some areas of Worcestershire were beginning to open again. For some schools the opening was tinged with sorrow. The logbook of Ombersley School carried the following statement: 'Sorry to record the death of James Masdell (scholar) from the influenza.' Some schools seemed determined to carry on regardless, determined to maintain their traditions whatever the risk to their pupils. An irate parent wrote to the editor of the *Evening Dispatch* on 7 December 1918 complaining that the girls at King Edward's School in Camp Hill in Birmingham were expected to turn up wearing white muslin for their prize distribution in December, despite the influenza pandemic.

As Worcestershire was coming through the worst of the epidemic, Staffordshire schoolchildren were succumbing to it. The logbooks for Bilston Primary School demonstrate how children's education was interrupted. The school was closed for two weeks for the first time on 18 November 1918, on instructions from the County Medical Officer. They opened again on 2 December but only 85 out of 150 children on the registers were actually present. A week later the school was again closed until after Christmas. Even when the school reopened in January it struggled with attendance and sometimes 30-40% of the children were absent as a result of the final wave of influenza in

CHAPTER SEVEN

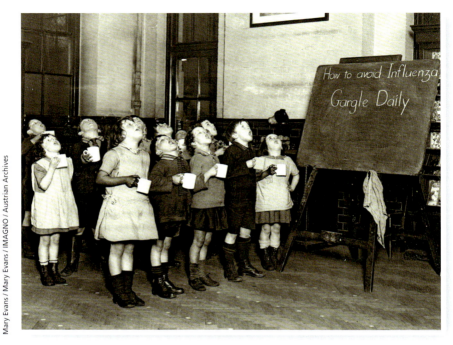

Little schoolchildren gargling their throats as a precaution against the influenza epidemic in England, c 1935.

February and March. In the Cannock district, at the end of November, the Education Committee learnt that 1,500 children were absent from school daily at the end of November 1918, and the average attendance was down by 20% - some of the children were ill, others had influenza in their family and in other cases parents kept them away from school, fearful they would catch influenza. One in six deaths in the region was a child of school age.

Closing schools did not prevent fatalities amongst either the pupils or their families. The Alice Ottley School in Worcester recorded in its history that there were several fatalities from the influenza, whilst Ethel Brown (née Robinson) who was aged only 9 and living in Coventry during the epidemic recalled:

> *I was one of a very large family of nine children ranging from 10 months to 15 years of age. Eight of the family went down with the flu including my mother, doctors called in twice a day. I was the only one of the family that didn't have the virus. Therefore I was doing my best*

to help the others. Of course no-one else would come into the house owing to so many of my family being so ill with the flu. After a few days some of my brothers and sisters were able to get up and help but when we had five of the family still sick my sister aged 7 years old died, November 3rd then on November 5th my mother died... my mother only at the age of 35. It caused quite a sensation having a double funeral, which was on November 11th 1918, which was the day the First World War ended. I can remember very well when the cortège was on its way to the Church bell hooters and all sounds of celebration were raving but how silent people stood who realized it was our funeral. It really was a terrible time not knowing who we were going to lose next. The doctor said afterwards he expected to sign five death certificates in our family everyone was so ill.

A number of children became orphans, many children lost their mothers in the epidemic; one in eight of the women who became war widows during the First World War died within a year of their husbands. Influenza contributed to this statistic, and its ability to sweep through families hit children hard. Mr and Mrs W. Clarke of Norton Bridge, Staffordshire, died within a few days of each other in December 1918: the young couple were both under 30 years of age. They left three young children, the youngest of whom was not yet ten weeks old. In Badsey Mrs Winford died after she attended the wedding of a relative in Evesham before she had properly recovered from influenza: she developed pneumonia. She left her husband a widower with nine children to care for. Although the end of December brought some respite in the flu, for some children and their families the tragedy continued. The *Evesham Journal* reported on 14 December 1918 that Mr and Mrs T. Hands in Cherington, instead of preparing to celebrate the approaching Christmas festivities with their youngsters, had to bury all their three small children. The little mites were aged 5 and 4 years and their baby was only 11 months old; they all died of whooping cough and influenza.

At the end of 1918, many teachers may have hoped that they had seen the last of influenza, with the head at Suckley, Worcestershire, noting in his log that 'it has been the worst period I have known.... Work and poor staff through illness, closure through cough'. But in February and March the third wave of

CHAPTER SEVEN

influenza arrived and with it chaos, teacher illness and school closures once again. Astley Church of England School, Worcestershire, closed from 26 February to 10 March, having already lost a month of school in November. The head teacher of Biddulph Primary School in Staffordshire recorded in the logbook for March 1919, once again, that attendance was low because of the prevalence of influenza. He seemed exasperated by the number of parents whose children did not have influenza but were being kept off school as a precautionary measure and by the absence of one of the teachers for nearly two weeks. Across the region the news was the same; children were ill with influenza and bronchitis in Ombersley in Worcestershire. In Shipston-on-Stour Girl Guides formed a guard of honour at the funeral of one of their number. Hilda Agnes Nellie Dyer died in February 1919 aged just 18.

CHAPTER EIGHT

Afterword: loss, legacies and futures

The greatest legacy of influenza for most people in the West Midlands was the loss not only of their loved ones and friends but also of their hopes and dreams for families and communities in the post-war world that were snatched away by the death of parent, spouse or fiancé. Many families, like that of Wilfred Mason Brooks who had lived in the Croft, Finstall near Bromsgrove until his death in December 1918, were devastated by influenza. Wilfred left a wife and three children, the youngest only three weeks old suffering, like her mother, from flu. Influenza stole the happy-ever-after ending from so many couples. Lieutenant Fredrick Thurston Stringer, the only son of parents who lived in Bredon, Worcestershire, had been educated in Malvern and Gosport, Hampshire before going to Dartmouth Naval College where he passed his Royal Naval Cadetship. Two years later, after passing his final examination, he became a midshipman on *H.M.S. Albion* and then went on to command *H.M.S. Weir*. He married his fiancée Miss Tyl in June 1918 but died of complications from influenza in Plymouth in April 1919, before their life together had really begun.

Other families never came into being. In Worcestershire two young women died on what should have been their wedding day; others died while still looking forward to their 'big day'. Miss Ethel Hawker was the youngest daughter and during the war the 'right hand' of her father, a dairyman in Evesham. Ethel had taken on the role of delivering milk in the town for her father, when her brother joined the army. Later in the summer of 1918 she became engaged to Sergeant W. E. Cartwright of the Royal Field Artillery whose father was also a dairyman. However, on returning from a fortnight's holiday, Ethel was ill for nine days, initially with influenza, but then she contracted pneumonia and died, just shy of her twenty-fifth birthday and just before her fiancé was due home on leave.

For many widows, widowers and orphans, when the Spanish flu killed a loved one it was not only an emotional loss but also precipitated a financial crisis as families struggled to survive prior to the welfare state. For those whose husbands died of influenza whilst still serving in the armed forces, the newly-introduced War Widow's Pension, a regular payment, received as of right rather than having to rely on charity, stood between them and penury. Corporal James Jones whose parents lived in Halt Heath, Worcestershire, was, as a member of the Yeomanry, mobilised in 1914. He sustained injuries in the arm and back during the Battle of Somme but after five months recovering in a French hospital, died of influenza after four days of illness on 2 November 1918. His wife and parents may not have been informed of his death before the Armistice. His one child would grow up fatherless, but his wife would at least have received a £5 death grant for herself and an additional £1 for their child. As he died on active service, his wife was also eligible for the War Widow's Pension. She would have received 16 shillings and 8d (83 pence) a week for herself and 6 shillings and 8 d (33 pence) a week for her child, although this would be reduced when her child turned 16. She would continue to receive her pension for the rest of her life as long as she did not re-marry or behave in any way that was considered 'inappropriate'. She was one of the lucky ones: many servicemen's wives were not. George Whatcott of Chipping Campden had joined the Royal Field Artillery in 1916 and served in France for 12 months before he was finally demobilised in February 1919. On his journey back to Britain he appeared to have caught a cold and when he arrived home on 8 February he felt ill and went to bed. Despite visits from the doctor he died on 16 February from double pneumonia, following influenza. His wife would not have been eligible for War Widow's Pension, as his death occurred technically after he was released from the armed forces.

Widow's pensions were not introduced more widely until the Widows, Orphans and Old Age Contributors Act of 1925, too late for the widow of Roger Webley, a boot maker from 36 High Street, Bromsgrove, who died of pleurisy and pneumonia within two weeks of catching influenza in November 1918. He had been in the Machine Gun Section of the Bromsgrove Volunteers, and an active member of the local football club. However, the future would have looked particularly bleak for his wife, who the newspapers described as 'crippled' and who would have received no widow's pension and was likely to have been reliant on charity and what work she could manage. She was left with six children, the eldest of whom was nine, and trying and find a way to support her family would have been very difficult. Little wonder that in such circumstances many women gave their children into the care either of other members of their

CHAPTER EIGHT

family if they were lucky, or to charities like Dr Barnardo's if they were not. Indeed influenza may well have been a significant stimulus for the 1925 Act which introduced both widow's pensions and the first bereavement or death payments to help cover funeral costs. The epidemic may also have further spurred other social reforms, for example, increasing the impetus towards more infant and maternal welfare. However, in the economic crisis of the inter-war years progress was slow.

The misguided assumption that influenza was a consequence of dirt and bacteria, particularly in inner city areas such as Birmingham and Stoke-on-Trent or Coventry, added weight to a number of prominent political campaigns for social change in the inter-war years. 'Homes fit for Heroes' was a key campaign slogan of the first post-war general election on 14 December 1918. This election, fought against the background of the second most fatal wave of influenza, was

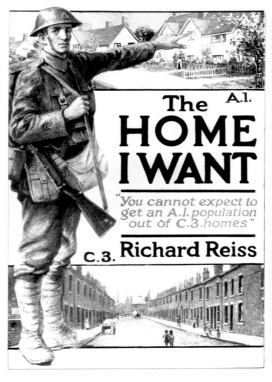

Housing poster, 'The Home I Want', with a quotation from Richard Reiss: 'You cannot expect to get an A.1.population out of C.3.homes'. The poster depicts a soldier returning from war and aspiring to live in a better environment.

also the election in which all men and those women who were over thirty and met the property qualifications could vote for the first time. The 'Homes Fit for Heroes' slogan appealed to both men and women and addressed the immediate needs of many of the new voters. Many believed, despite evidence to the contrary, that the poor state of housing had contributed to the spread of influenza. When Dr Robertson, the Medical Officer for Health in Birmingham, came to write his annual report for 1918, he attributed the high mortality rates from influenza to inadequate knowledge of how the infection spread and also to the deficient state of housing. This was a view held not only in Birmingham but also in the Gloucestershire town of Tewkesbury, which had got off lightly in terms of fatalities from influenza by comparison with Birmingham. The *Cheltenham Chronicle and Gloucestershire Graphic* reported on 2 November 1918 the view of campaigners who, when discussing influenza, suggested: 'To those who know the hovels in which the sufferers are doomed to live, it is cause for wonder that fatal results have not been more numerous'. The newspaper suggested that such housing needed burning down and replacing.

There was in some areas of the West Midlands a political will to address the housing problem and new Labour members of West Bromwich Council, who in December 1918 numbered four, campaigned strongly for early action on the housing question. The *Evening Dispatch* reported on 5 December 1918 that a councillor, using influenza as a reference point, had argued: 'many lives could have been saved by proper air, space and proper housing' and that house-building had the added benefit of providing employment for demobbed men. In 1919, Parliament passed a Housing Act, which promised government subsidies to help finance the construction of 500,000 houses by 1922. Dr Robertson, the Medical Officer for Health in Birmingham, noted that:

> *It is true that much discussion has taken place and that a new Act of Parliament has been passed fixing greatly extended powers for building and reconstruction. The new houses, which are in contemplation will relieve the grievous overcrowding, but will not do anything to solve our slum problem.*

In April 1919, Kidderminster Rural District was likewise busy discussing the housing problem and the need for the issue of 'slumdom' in urban and rural

CHAPTER EIGHT

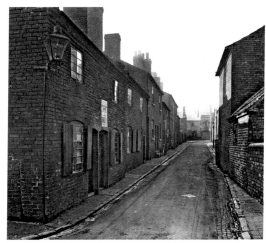

A photograph of the terraced houses in Hall Street, Tipton, prior to slum clearance, c.1930.

Photograph Courtesy of Sandwell Community History and Archives Service, PHS/917

areas to be addressed. However, the economic straits that Britain found itself in during the 1920s and 1930s meant that the abolition of slums and building of new affordable homes was slow and patchy. It was an area of political activity for many feminist and women's groups at national and local levels who put housing high on their agendas, a prioritisation which was arguably stimulated by the Spanish flu.

On 28 June 1919 the Treaty of Versailles was signed, finally marking the end of the First World War. When the peace parades and celebrations were held in the months that followed, most of Britain at least had seen the end of the influenza pandemic, but not of the fear and anxieties that the pandemic created. As the war was ending, some doctors, such as Arthur Sladden from Badsey in Worcestershire, had already identified the need to change healthcare. Writing to his sister in November 1918, he remarked:

> *I hope this influenza epidemic will do good in one way, in leading to a proper co-ordination of preventative medicine – and yet I have doubts, we are essentially a "wait and see" nation.... So if a Ministry of Health or a State Medical Service is formed, we shan't necessarily get much further unless they get very good men in control.*

Influenza, and a good deal of political manoeuvring, did lead to the setting up of a Ministry of Health in 1919. However, when George Newman at the

CHAPTER EIGHT

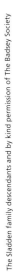

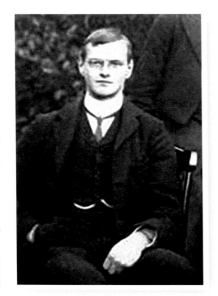

Andrew Sladden, a military doctor from Worcestershire who hoped the pandemic would lead to the setting up of a Ministry of Health

Ministry of Health delivered his 'Report on the Pandemic of Influenza 1918-9' to Christopher Addison MD, MP and Minister of Health, he had to acknowledge that 'the problem of influenza is still unsolved' and its solution, he suggested, would be 'one of the great events in the history of medicine'. He went on to explain that the global outlook regarding future pestilences or the dangers of pestilence was gloomy. In the meantime, the report suggested some administrative reorganisation and many of the suggestions that had been unsuccessful in combating the virus over the previous eighteen months were also repeated.

> Firstly we must fortify our administrative methods for dealing with such scourges as influenza, and secondly, we must instruct the whole population, child and adult in the laws of preventive medicine…
>
> Avoid overcrowding and thronging of every sort, whether in places of public resort, public conveyances, or factories. Well-ventilated rooms, nourishing food and an open-air life afford some defence… At the first feeling of illness, or rise in temperature it is the private and public duty of the patient to go to bed at once, to remain at rest and in warmth, and to place himself under medical supervision, for it cannot be too clearly understood that it is the complications of influenza which disable or destroy life.

A century later, there are very different administrative structures and importantly a National Health Service providing medical care for all. The flu vaccination which many people have in the autumn is one of the main preventive

CHAPTER EIGHT

measures taken to avoid catching the disease. However, there is still speculation as to whether another influenza pandemic could cause death and destruction on the same scale as that seen between 1918 and 1920. Such speculation is encouraged by science fiction and disaster movies such as *Contagion* (2011) or *The Flu* (2013) which was produced in South Korea.

Influenza viruses can be thought of as simple, self-replicating machines, containing the bare minimum of genetic information needed to infect humans. They comprise of just eight segments of genetic material, compared to the 20,000 or so genes which humans have. Influenza viruses take over human cells in order to make copies of themselves, but do so very inaccurately. On average, they make one mistake per new virus: it is these mistakes which can lead to changes in their external structure, making them unrecognisable to a person's immune system.

The human immune system is very efficient at getting rid of viruses it has come across before but because the flu virus keeps changing, it is more difficult for the human immune system to respond strongly. That is why people keep getting flu. When small changes are involved, some people will still be immune to the virus, because their immune system recognises a structure that essentially has not changed. However, when a virus that is radically different from the previously circulating virus enters the human population - sometimes because it has swapped some genes with an animal influenza virus, or is itself an animal virus - nobody has any pre-existing immunity. This is what causes pandemics.

Radically different viruses will appear again, and be capable of infecting huge numbers of people, as happened in 1918. However, the world today is a very different place, and global travel is much more common, and much more rapid. Transatlantic travel is achieved in a matter of hours rather than taking a week. People live in cities of ever increasing size, and utilise methods of mass transportation that squeeze thousands of people into close proximity, and importantly within the six-foot radius across which flu spreads from one person to another. It can be safely assumed that any new virus could spread much more quickly than the 1918 pandemic. This could have the potential to cause a similar number of deaths as in 1918, but this would probably happen almost simultaneously around the globe.

However, there are reasons for optimism, especially for those lucky enough to be born in a wealthy country with an established public health system. Deaths in flu pandemics are frequently due to secondary, bacterial infections. There are now ranges of antibiotics to help prevent these infections becoming fatal. Bacteria are rapidly evolving resistance to antibiotics, so more research is necessary to develop new varieties. However, those of us who live in the twenty-first century are significantly better placed in this regard than the population of 1918. There are also two anti-influenza drugs available, with more in the pipeline, and other pharmacological options for treating flu. One of these drugs has been shown to be effective against the 1918 strain. There are also better ways of helping people to absorb enough oxygen into their bodies when their lungs are damaged. A report in 1920 suggested that if enough oxygen could be got into patients, then they might have had a chance of surviving the infection. These options are not available to most of the world's population; they are expensive, due at least in part to the huge amount of research invested in their design and testing.

The sad truth is that much of the world's population is at just as much risk from pandemic flu now as they have ever been. Only a global strategy will protect everyone. This is difficult for influenza because it has animal hosts. It is not like the smallpox virus, which has no non-human hosts, and was successfully eradicated with mass vaccination in the 1970s; one of the most brilliant examples of human cooperation in history. Flu cannot be eradicated from humans because they keep catching it from animals. Nevertheless, vaccination might still provide a solution. Seasonal flu vaccines change every year, depending on which viruses are found to be circulating by a global network of laboratories and scientists. These vaccines trigger an immune response to components of the virus that change over time. They are currently the best weapon against seasonal flu, but they take a long time to produce, and new ones have to be produced every year. For seasonal flu, scientists have 8 months between deciding which strains the vaccine should protect against, and producing a sufficient quantity of it to protect the population. Were a new pandemic virus to emerge, this luxury would not exist. What is needed is a cheap and effective 'universal flu vaccine', that is a vaccine that could protect people against any potential flu virus, by generating an immune response against a part of the virus that does not keep changing. This is the 'Holy Grail' of influenza research. Such vaccines are currently undergoing trials by a number of research groups around the world. Only time will tell whether it will be successful but scientists are optimistic about its chances.

Sources

As well as newspapers, this book has drawn upon and quoted from the following archival and online sources:

Badsey History Society, Letter from Arthur Sladden to his sister in November 1918 https://www.badseysociety.uk/sladden-archive/letters/afss19181102

https://birminghamhistory.co.uk/forum/index.php?threads/spanish-flu-epidemic-in-birmingham.33886/

Birmingham Museum, Hilda Moss of 65 Streetly Lane, Four Oaks, Sutton Coldfield, Birmingham, interview undertaken on 10 August 1981

Cadbury Research Centre, *The Mermaid*, November 1918, UB/GUILD/F/3/17 The Mermaid Folder, Number 4 & 5

https://www.florence-nightingale.co.uk/wp-content/uploads/2018/11/Secondary-Resource-Pack-LR.pdf

Birmingham Archives, Colin Priestman's letter to his mother. Letter 25 June 1918, MS 327 /A /1 /65

Hereford Archives Service, Ruth Bourne Diaries 1913-1919. The First World War. AK22/47.

Staffordshire Archives, Record of the experiences of Lance-Corporal John Henry Turner, 1914-1918. D1549. Staffordshire Record Office.

Wellcome Library, Medical Officer of Health Reports https://wellcomelibrary.org/moh/about-the-reports/about-the-medical-officer-of-health-reports/

Wolfson Centre, Birmingham, Letter from Cyril Cartwright to Gertie Cartwright, MS 2682/2/1

Further Reading

Andrews, Margaret W. "Epidemic and Public Health: Influenza in Vancouver, 1918-1919." BC Studies: *The British Columbian Quarterly* 34 (1977): 21-44.

Arnold, Catharine. *Pandemic 1918: The Story of the Deadliest Influenza in History*. Michael O'Mara Books, 2018.

Collier, Richard. *The Plague of the Spanish Lady: The Influenza Pandemic of 1918-1919*. New York: Atheneum, 1974.

Cox, Francis. *World War: Disease, The Only Victor*. https://www.gresham.ac.uk/lectures-and-events/the-first-world-war-disease-the-only-victor#tRD2o4G5wFxqzjyK.99

Duncan, Kirsty. *Hunting the 1918 Flu: One Scientist's Search for a Killer Virus*. University of Toronto Press, 2003.

Honigsbaum, Mark. *Living with Enza: The Forgotten Story of Britain and the Great Flu Pandemic of 1918*. Springer, 2016.

Hume, Robert. "When Spanish Flu came to Britain". *BBC History Magazine*, 28 December 2017. https://www.pressreader.com/uk/bbc-history-magazine/20171228/283321817743897

Johnson, Niall. *Britain and the 1918-19 Influenza Pandemic: A Dark Epilogue*. Routledge, 2006.

Restifo, Nicholas P. "Flu: The Story of the Great Influenza Pandemic of 1918 and the Search for the Virus that Caused it." *Nature Medicine* 2000; 6:12-13.

Spinney, Laura. *Pale Rider: The Spanish Flu of 1918 and How it Changed the World*. Public Affairs, 2017.

Winter, Jay. *The Great War and the British People*. Springer, 2003.

World Heath Organization https://www.who.int/influenza

INDEX

Alcohol (and alcoholism and drinking) 26, 30, 50, 51, 52–53, 63, 67

Armistice 33, 37, 38, 39, 64, 65, 75, 84, 93, 94, 100

Babies (see also infant welfare) 70, 87, 88, 89, 97

Bacteria 11, 12, 15, 16, 17, 26, 45, 63, 92, 101, 105, 106

Badsey 28, 29, 64, 97, 103, 104

Birmingham 5, 7, 8, 10, 12, 13, 14, 15, 16, 19, 20, 22, 24, 25, 27, 31, 32, 33, 34, 35, 36, 38, 39, 44, 45, 46, 47, 49, 52, 55, 56, 58, 60, 61, 63, 64, 65, 66, 68, 71, 73, 75, 76, 77, 78, 79, 80, 81, 82, 83, 84, 85, 86, 87, 89, 90, 91, 93, 94, 95, 101, 102

Black Country 7, 24, 38, 49

Bovril 51, 53-55, 54-57

Bromsgrove 13, 29, 37, 38, 49, 51, 70, 88, 99, 100

Burton-on-Trent 8, 74, 77

Cannock Chase 19, 24, 37, 66, 96

Catarrh 22, 26, 64

Cemeteries 34, 37, 77, 80, 84

Chamberlain family 34, 35

Chemists 53, 58, 60

Children 35, 39, 45, 47, 50, 59, 61, 70, 71, 73, 75, 76, 86-98, 99, 100

Chinese Labour Corps 15

Cinemas / picture houses 6, 7, 32, 45, 46, 47

Clergy 76-77, 86-7

Coventry 7, 12, 20, 35, 36, 48, 60, 68, 77, 84, 96, 101

Dirt 19, 21, 27, 84, 92, 101

Disinfectant 17, 21, 32, 45

Doctors 6, 11, 12, 16, 17, 18, 22, 24, 30, 31, 36, 39, 40, 44, 50, 52, 54, 56-72, 96, 103

Dr Williams Pink Pills for Pale People 43-44

Droitwich 29, 51, 59

Dudley 38, 49, 69-70, 93

Evesham (and Evesham Vale) 8, 13, 19, 28, 29, 30, 31, 46, 54, 70, 71, 75, 79, 88, 97, 99

Factories 6, 7, 8, 13, 24, 28, 31, 32, 54, 67, 77, 89, 104

Families 6, 7, 13, 19, 24, 25, 27, 28, 33, 34, 44, 48, 50, 51, 53, 67, 69, 70, 71, 75, 77, 78, 80, 81, 82, 84, 85, 93, 96, 97, 99, 100, 101, 104

Fladbury 8

Food shortages and malnutrition 7, 8, 16, 19, 23, 28, 29, 30, 34, 53-55, 70, 76, 80, 104

109

INDEX

Football 45, 100

Funerals 8, 29, 34, 49, 73, 75-82, 84, 85, 93, 97, 98, 101

Gargling 17, 47, 96

Germany and Germans 7, 8, 15, 16, 28

Herefordshire 7, 49, 50, 60

Hospitals (and infirmaries) 9, 28, 32, 40, 41, 64-67, 70, 71, 75, 100

Housewives 7, 29, 69, 70, 73

Housing 19, 27, 101-103

Infant Welfare 68, 87-88

Kidderminster 8, 13, 19, 20, 31, 34, 49, 65, 74, 76, 77, 87, 94, 102,

Local government (including district councils) 16, 24, 51, 61, 67, 71, 84, 88,

Malvern 33, 48, 63, 65, 76, 88, 93, 99,

Manufacturing 7, 28, 30, 32, 42, 44, 52, 57

Measles 22

Medical Officers of Health 5, 12, 14, 16, 22, 24, 25, 26, 31, 34, 36, 44, 45, 46, 47, 55, 63, 70, 92, 93, 94, 95, 102

Mines (and miners) 7, 13, 24, 59

Munitions 7, 13, 24, 33, 59, 73, 77

Nurses (and nursing) 22, 40, 64, 65-71, 73, 88, 93

Orphans 86, 97, 99, 100

Pauper's funeral 78, 80, 85

Pensions 85, 100, 101

Pershore 13, 29, 47, 49

Pfeiffer's bacillus 16, 17

Medicals (including staff, profession, service, students and experts) 17, 18, 20, 21, 24, 27, 40, 41, 50, 51, 56, 57, 58, 59, 60, 63, 64, 65

Pneumonia 9, 22, 24, 27, 28, 30, 36, 37, 40, 42, 47, 49, 50, 51, 61. 64, 66, 67, 71, 76, 88, 89, 93, 97, 99, 100

Police (and courts) 19, 34, 42, 61, 70, 75, 76, 94

Poverty 27, 30, 78

POW (Prisoner of War) 9, 19, 28, 29, 37, 38, 39

Prevention (of influenza) 53, 56, 67, 69, 71, 72

Public transport (also see trains) 8, 22, 47

Queues 6, 7, 58

Royal Army Medical Corps (RAMC) 18, 20

Russian Flu 6, 13, 15, 22, 35, 42, 53

Schools 6, 8, 14, 19, 20, 22, 44, 45, 46, 49, 56, 76, 86-98

Scientists 17, 61, 106

INDEX

Shops and stores 35, 50, 51, 53, 54, 73, 76

Smoking 24, 74

Soldiers and armed forces 8, 9, 12, 15, 20, 38, 54, 56, 57, 59, 64, 65, 73, 78, 84, 87, 88, 89, 99, 100,

Spain 6, 57

Stafford 7, 16

Staffordshire 7, 15, 24, 33, 37, 41, 49, 65, 67, 76, 95, 97, 98

Stoke-on-Trent (including the Potteries) 24, 31, 39, 41, 49, 88, 101

Stourport 13, 31

Stourbridge 49, 67

Teachers 22, 73, 76, 89, 93, 94, 95, 97, 98

Tewkesbury 102

Theatres (including music halls) 8, 32, 45, 46

Trains / railways 9, 28, 40, 70, 74, 75,

Undertakers (including funeral directors) 6, 36, 73, 78-82, 84

University 11, 33, 90-92

VAD (Voluntary Aid Detachment) 40, 41, 66-67, 71

Viruses 6, 8, 9, 10, 11-12, 15, 16-17, 18, 19, 20, 28, 33, 34, 37, 42, 45, 47, 49, 50, 56, 64, 65, 66, 68, 71, 86, 90, 92, 94, 95, 96, 104, 105, 106

Weddings (including marriage) 71, 77, 97, 99

West Bromwich 35, 75, 76, 82, 102

Whisky 50, 51-53

Widows (and widowers) 71, 75, 76, 85, 97, 99, 100, 101

Worcester 7, 13, 16, 21, 26, 27, 28, 30, 31, 34, 42, 45, 46, 60, 61, 63, 64, 65, 67, 69, 70, 76, 82, 86, 88, 89, 92, 93, 96

Worcestershire 8, 16, 20, 28, 29, 31, 33, 39, 47, 49, 60, 63, 70, 71, 79, 92, 93, 95, 97, 98, 99, 100, 103, 104

Workhouse 93, 95,

Wolverhampton 12, 45, 84, 93